DR. SEBI'S ALKALINE
AND ANTI-INFLAMMATORY DIET TRANSFORMATION FOR BEGINNERS

Discover Dr. Sebi's Path to Longevity by Mastering His Techniques and the Ultimate 28-Day Detox Plan

ROSALINDA MONTES

Dr. Sebi's Alkaline and Anti-Inflammatory Diet Transformation for Beginners

Discover Dr. Sebi's Path to Longevity by Mastering His Techniques and the Ultimate 28-Day Detox Plan

Copyright © 2023 by Rosalinda Montes

Printed in the United States of America

Thank You For Your Support!

★★★★★

I'm eager to know what you think!

Simply **scan this QR code** to jump straight to my book's review page on Amazon.

Your insights are invaluable – they aid in my growth as an author and assist others in discovering this book.

Feel free to **share a photo or video review showcasing you with the book**. Your experience could inspire others to embark on their adventure with my book!

Rosalinda

CONTENTS

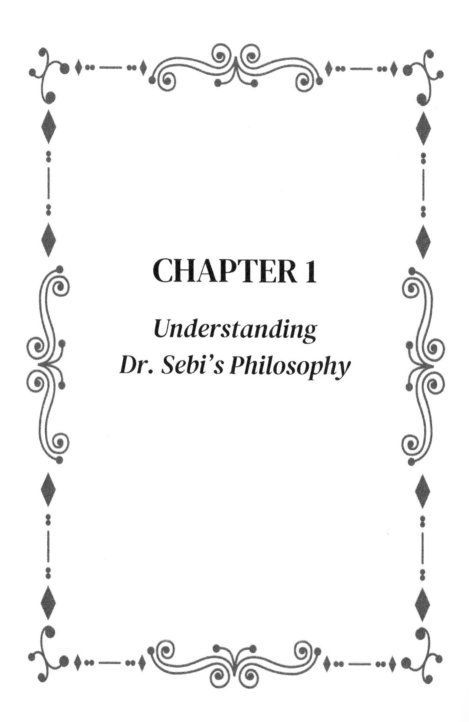

CHAPTER 1

Understanding Dr. Sebi's Philosophy

Who Was Dr. Sebi?

D r. Sebi, born Alfredo Darrington Bowman on November 26, 1933, in the small village of Ilanga in Honduras, had a humble beginning that played a significant role in shaping his later life and health philosophies. Raised in a rural setting, he was surrounded by nature and traditional ways of living. His grandmother, a traditional healer, and his mother, who valued natural remedies, influenced his early understanding of health and wellness. Despite the natural surroundings, Dr. Sebi's early life was not without its challenges, particularly regarding his health.

As a young man, Dr. Sebi faced numerous health struggles that would later fuel his quest for knowledge about natural healing. In his early twenties, after moving to the United States, he developed several chronic health issues, including obesity, diabetes, impotence, and asthma. These conditions were exacerbated by a standard American diet high in processed foods and low in nutritional value, which lacked the essential nutrients his body needed. Despite seeking help from conventional medicine, he found no relief, as treatments often focused on symptoms rather than addressing the root cause. This period of illness and frustration was a turning point for Dr. Sebi, motivating him to explore alternative methods of healing and eventually leading him to develop his own dietary philosophy centered around plant-based nutrition and herbal medicine.

Desperate for a solution, Dr. Sebi began exploring alternative approaches to health. He traveled extensively, learning from various traditional healing practices, including African herbalism, Ayurveda, and traditional Chinese medicine. During his travels, he encountered a Mexican herbalist who introduced him to the concept of a plant-based, alkaline diet. This meeting was pivotal; it sparked his lifelong dedication to natural healing and holistic health. Embracing this new approach, Dr. Sebi adopted a strict diet of natural, unprocessed foods and began using herbal remedies. He eliminated all animal products, refined sugars, and processed foods from his diet, focusing instead on consuming fruits, vegetables, nuts, seeds, and herbs. This dietary shift had a profound impact on his health. He experienced significant improvements in his chronic conditions, losing weight, gaining energy, and reversing his diabetes and impotence. These personal health transformations reinforced his belief in the power of natural healing and solidified his commitment to sharing this knowledge with others.

Dr. Sebi's early health struggles were instrumental in shaping his holistic health philosophy. They provided him with firsthand experience of the limitations of conventional medicine and the potential of natural remedies. His personal journey from illness to health became the foundation for his later work as a healer and herbalist. He dedicated his life to researching and developing natural healing protocols that emphasize the importance of an alkaline diet and the use of herbal medicine. Throughout his career, Dr. Sebi faced skepticism and criticism from the medical establishment, but his personal health journey and the testimonies of those he helped provided a powerful counter-narrative. His experiences underscored the importance of looking beyond conventional wisdom to explore alternative approaches to health and wellness.

Dr. Sebi's personal health struggles not only served as a catalyst for his transformation but also laid the groundwork for his lifelong mission to help others achieve wellness through natural means. After experiencing the profound effects of an alkaline, plant-based diet on his own health, Dr. Sebi became passionately committed to understanding the underlying principles that led to his recovery. This journey of discovery would eventually evolve into a comprehensive dietary and health philosophy that garnered a significant following worldwide.

Driven by curiosity and the desire to help others, Dr. Sebi began an extensive period of self-education and research. He immersed himself in the study of natural healing methods, focusing particularly on the medicinal properties of plants. He traveled to various parts of the world, learning from traditional healers and herbalists, and incorporating their wisdom into his own practice. This period of exploration and learning was crucial in developing his unique approach to health, which emphasized the importance of maintaining an alkaline internal environment to prevent disease.

During his studies, Dr. Sebi identified what he believed to be the root cause of many chronic illnesses: mucus buildup in the body. He theorized that the accumulation of mucus was a result of consuming acidic foods and that it was this mucus that obstructed the body's pathways, leading to disease. This concept became a cornerstone of his dietary philosophy, and he dedicated himself to educating others about the dangers of an acidic diet and the benefits of alkaline foods.

In the early 1980s, Dr. Sebi established the USHA Healing Village in Honduras, a wellness center where he could put his theories into practice and offer treatments to those seeking natural remedies for their ailments. At the USHA Village, he treated patients with a range of conditions, from chronic diseases like diabetes and hypertension to more severe illnesses such as HIV/AIDS and cancer. His approach involved a combination of dietary changes, herbal supplements, and natural therapies designed to cleanse the body of toxins and restore its natural balance. His initial success in treating patients at the USHA Village attracted attention and led to a growing reputation as a healer. People from around the world sought his advice and treatments, and many reported significant improvements in their health. Notably, high-profile individuals such as Michael Jackson, Lisa 'Left Eye' Lopes, John Travolta, Eddie Murphy, and Steven Seagal were among his clients. These testimonials from celebrities further solidified Dr. Sebi's belief in the efficacy of his methods and fueled his mission to spread the message of natural healing.

Despite his growing popularity, Dr. Sebi faced significant challenges from the medical establishment and regulatory authorities. His claims of curing diseases using natural methods were met with skepticism and legal challenges. In 1988, he was sued in New York for practicing medicine without a license. However, Dr. Sebi famously won the case by presenting testimony and evidence from patients who had been healed through his treatments. This legal victory bolstered his credibility and brought his methods to a wider audience.

Throughout his life, Dr. Sebi remained dedicated to educating others about the importance of diet and natural healing. He conducted lectures, wrote books, and produced educational materials to spread his message. His philosophy emphasized the importance of returning to natural, unprocessed foods and avoiding the artificial and processed products that dominate modern diets.

This book is designed to guide you on a journey towards better health through the principles of Dr. Sebi's alkaline diet. You'll find a comprehensive collection of recipes that adhere to his dietary guidelines, focusing on natural, nutrient-rich ingredients that promote healing and well-being. Expect practical advice on incorporating these foods into your daily life, along with tips for avoiding common dietary pitfalls. Whether you are new to Dr. Sebi's philosophy or looking to deepen your understanding, this book aims to be an invaluable resource for achieving and maintaining optimal health naturally.

Core Principles of Dr. Sebi's Dietary Theories

You must have gained a hint of Dr. Sebi's core philosophies from the preceding introduction. To recap, his dietary theories are grounded in the belief that maintaining an alkaline environment within the body is essential for optimal health and disease prevention. His philosophy emphasizes the consumption of natural, plant-based foods and the avoidance of processed, acidic foods. Here are the core principles of Dr. Sebi's dietary theories:

1. Alkalinity and pH Balance

Dr. Sebi posited that many diseases thrive in an acidic environment and that promoting an alkaline state within the body can create conditions that are less conducive to disease development. His theories suggest that eating alkaline-forming foods can produce a hostile environment for disease while also improving overall health. The pH scale, which ranges from 0 to 14, measures the acidity or alkalinity of a substance, with 7 being neutral. The human body naturally regulates its pH levels, especially in the blood, which maintains a slightly alkaline pH of around 7.35 to 7.45. Dr. Sebi argued that the modern diet, rich in processed foods, refined sugars, and animal products, tends to make the body more acidic. This acidic state, he believed, fosters an environment where the body contributes to the buildup of mucus and toxins. He theorized that mucus is a byproduct of the body's response to excess acidity and that this mucus buildup is a root cause of many diseases. For instance, conditions like respiratory issues, digestive problems, and even chronic illnesses like cancer are believed, in Dr. Sebi's view, to be exacerbated by an acidic internal environment. By reducing acidity and promoting alkalinity, the body can potentially prevent mucus buildup and reduce the risk of disease.

Consequently, Dr. Sebi recommended avoiding acid-forming foods, which he believed contribute to an acidic internal environment. These foods include processed foods, refined sugars, artificial sweeteners, caffeine, alcohol, and animal products like meat and dairy. Processed foods, in particular, are seen as detrimental due to their high content of preservatives, additives, and lack of essential nutrients. Eliminating these foods from your diet can help to reduce your body's acidity and promote a more alkaline condition.

2. Natural, Plant-Based Diet

Dr. Sebi was a staunch advocate of a natural, plant-based diet, emphasizing the consumption of foods that are as close to their natural state as possible. This dietary approach prioritizes fruits, vegetables, nuts, seeds, and grains, which Dr. Sebi believed were inherently more beneficial for the body compared to processed foods. He argued that plant-based diets, rich in essential nutrients, support the body's natural detoxification processes and overall health. He maintained that these foods, unaltered by industrial processes, retain their nutritional integrity and provide the body with the vitamins, minerals, and antioxidants necessary for optimal health. According to Dr. Sebi, the consumption of plant-based foods helps to prevent the accumulation of toxins and mucus, which he believed were the underlying causes of many diseases.

From a traditional nutritional perspective, a natural, plant-based diet is rich in a variety of nutrients that support overall health. Fruits and vegetables provide essential vitamins such as vitamin C, vitamin A, and folate, as well as minerals like potassium and magnesium. These nutrients play crucial roles in maintaining bodily functions, from supporting the immune system to promoting healthy skin and vision. Nuts and seeds, another key component of Dr. Sebi's diet, are excellent sources of healthy fats, protein, and fiber. They contain essential fatty acids like omega-3s, which are important for brain health and reducing inflammation. Whole grains such as quinoa, brown rice, and oats offer complex carbohydrates and fiber, providing sustained energy and aiding in digestion. The high fiber content in fruits, vegetables, nuts, seeds, and grains helps to promote regular bowel movements, which is crucial for the elimination of toxins from the body. Additionally, the antioxidants found in plant-based foods help to neutralize free radicals, reducing oxidative stress and the risk of chronic diseases.

3. Avoidance of Processed and Acidic Foods

Processed foods are those that have been altered from their natural state through various methods, including canning, freezing, refrigeration, dehydration, and aseptic processing. These foods often contain artificial additives, preservatives, colorings, and flavorings, which Dr. Sebi believed were harmful to the body. He argued that the consumption of these foods leads to an imbalance in the body's pH levels, creating an acidic environment that promotes the growth of disease-causing agents.

Refined sugars and white flour, common ingredients in processed foods, are stripped of their natural nutrients during the refining process. This leaves them as empty calories, contributing to weight gain, insulin resistance, and other metabolic disorders. Dr. Sebi asserted that these refined carbohydrates are particularly detrimental because they spike blood sugar levels, leading to inflammation and an acidic bodily environment.

Dairy products and meat are primary examples of acidic foods that Dr. Sebi recommended avoiding. Dairy products, although rich in calcium, are also high in lactose and casein, which can contribute to mucus production and inflammation. Similarly, meat, particularly red and processed meats, is acidic and can lead to the accumulation of uric acid in the body. This can exacerbate conditions like gout and kidney stones, and contribute to a general acidic state.

Artificial additives in food, such as preservatives, flavor enhancers, and colorings, are chemicals that the body does not naturally recognize. Dr. Sebi believed that these substances contribute to the body's toxin load, burdening the liver and other detoxification organs. Over time, the accumulation of these toxins can lead to chronic health issues and disrupt the body's natural processes.

4. Herbal Supplements

Dr. Sebi's health philosophy extended beyond diet to include herbal supplements designed to detoxify, enhance circulation, and support vital organ health. He believed these supplements helped cleanse the body of toxins and maintain a balanced internal environment, promoting overall well-being.

Key Supplements:

- **Bio Ferro:** Boosts iron levels, supports blood health, increases energy, improves circulation, and combats anemia.
- **Viento:** Provides natural energy, supports mental clarity, enhances physical performance, and aids in detoxification.
- **Chelation:** Removes heavy metals and toxins, cleanses blood and tissues, and supports organ function.
- **Sea Moss:** Rich in minerals like iodine and calcium, supports thyroid health, boosts the immune system, and aids in digestion and detoxification.
- **Banju:** Enhances brain and nervous system health, improves cognitive function, memory, and reduces stress.

5. The Importance of Hydration

Hydration is a cornerstone of Dr. Sebi's dietary principles, emphasizing the critical role of water and herbal teas in maintaining health and supporting the body's natural detoxification processes. Proper hydration helps flush out toxins, keeping the body's internal environment clean and balanced. Dr. Sebi specifically advocated for the consumption of natural spring water due to its mineral content and alkalizing properties, which help maintain the body's optimal pH levels.

Water is essential for various bodily functions, including digestion and nutrient absorption. Adequate hydration ensures that digestive enzymes function efficiently, aiding in the breakdown and assimilation of nutrients from food. Furthermore, water is crucial for the elimination of waste products through urine, sweat, and feces, preventing the buildup of toxins that can lead to disease.

Herbal teas also play a significant role in Dr. Sebi's hydration recommendations. Teas made from herbs like burdock root, dandelion, and ginger not only provide hydration but also offer additional health benefits, such as enhanced liver function, improved digestion, and anti-inflammatory effects.

In essence, staying well-hydrated with pure, natural liquids supports overall health, enhances detoxification, and aligns with Dr. Sebi's vision of a balanced, disease-free body.

6. Minimalism and Simplicity

Dr. Sebi's dietary philosophy strongly emphasizes minimalism and simplicity, advocating for a return to consuming foods in their most natural, unprocessed states. He believed that the human body operates optimally when it is not overloaded with the toxins and additives commonly found in processed foods. This minimalist approach involves selecting foods that are closer to their original form, such as fresh fruits, vegetables, nuts, seeds, and whole grains. Avoiding complex meals that require extensive processing or include artificial ingredients helps reduce the burden on the body's digestive and detoxification systems. Dr. Sebi asserted that a simplified diet not only promotes better digestion and nutrient absorption but also supports the body's natural ability to maintain a balanced pH and robust immune function.

7. Regular Fasting

Regular fasting is a key component of Dr. Sebi's dietary theories, rooted in the belief that periodic fasting aids in detoxification and the rejuvenation of the body. Dr. Sebi posited that fasting allows the digestive system to rest, thereby enabling the body to divert energy towards healing and eliminating accumulated waste products. This process can help cleanse the body of toxins, reduce inflammation, and support overall health.

Dr. Sebi recommended incorporating regular fasting into one's routine to enhance the body's natural healing processes. During fasting, the body is thought to undergo a sort of "reset," where it can more effectively manage and eliminate harmful substances that contribute to disease. This practice is aligned with the broader principle of minimalism and simplicity in his dietary approach, emphasizing the importance of giving the body time and space to heal without the constant influx of food and potential toxins.

8. Food Combining

Dr. Sebi placed significant emphasis on the importance of proper food combining, a concept that revolves around the idea that certain foods, when eaten together, can either enhance or hinder digestion and nutrient absorption. According to Dr. Sebi, improper food combinations can lead to digestive issues, decreased nutrient uptake, and increased toxin accumulation in the body.

For instance, Dr. Sebi suggested that starches and proteins should not be consumed in the same meal. He argued that these food groups require different digestive environments: proteins need an acidic environment, while starches require a more alkaline one. Consuming them together can slow down digestion and cause fermentation and bloating. Instead, he recommended pairing proteins with non-starchy vegetables and combining starches with other vegetables to facilitate smoother digestion.

Additionally, fruits should generally be eaten alone or with other fruits because they digest quickly and can ferment if mixed with slower-digesting foods. Following these meal combining principles can help you optimize your digestive processes, reduce gastrointestinal pain, and enhance overall nutrient absorption. This approach aligns with Dr. Sebi's broader dietary philosophy of maintaining a balanced and alkaline internal environment to promote health and prevent disease.

9. Electrical Foods

Dr. Sebi introduced the concept of "electrical foods," which he described as natural, non-hybrid foods that are rich in nutrients and high in energy. According to Dr. Sebi, these foods help "electrify" the body, providing it with the necessary vitality to function optimally and support overall health. Electrical foods are believed to align with the body's natural bioelectricity, promoting cellular health and efficiency.

Examples of electrical foods include a variety of fresh fruits, vegetables, nuts, seeds, and grains that have not been genetically modified or hybridized. Specific foods often highlighted in Dr. Sebi's diet include sea moss, nopal cactus, avocados, wild rice, and various leafy greens such as kale. These foods are chosen for their high mineral content, particularly in trace minerals that are crucial for bodily functions but often deficient in modern diets.

In juxtaposition, hybrid foods are those created by cross-breeding two different plant species to produce a new variety with specific desired traits. While these hybrid foods can offer benefits such as increased yield, improved resistance to pests, and enhanced flavor, Dr. Sebi contended that they are nutritionally inferior and potentially harmful to the body.

One of the primary concerns Dr. Sebi had with hybrid foods is their potential lack of nutritional integrity. He argued that hybridization often results in foods that are less nutritionally dense compared to their wild or original counterparts. According to Dr. Sebi, the natural genetic makeup of original plants, which has evolved over millennia, is optimal for human consumption. He believed that tampering with these genetics through hybridization could disrupt the delicate balance of nutrients, enzymes, and minerals that our bodies need to function properly.

Dr. Sebi also posited that hybrid foods could contribute to the buildup of mucus in the body, which he believed to be the root cause of many diseases. He suggested that these foods are more likely to be acidic and create an environment within the body that is conducive to mucus production. This viewpoint aligns with his broader dietary recommendation to consume alkaline foods that help maintain a slightly alkaline pH in the body, promoting overall health and preventing disease.

Moreover, Dr. Sebi was concerned about the potential long-term health effects of consuming hybrid foods. He theorized that because hybrid foods are often cultivated for traits like size, taste, and resilience rather than nutritional value, they might lack the necessary elements to support robust health. He emphasized the importance of consuming electric foods – those that are naturally grown, non-hybrid, and alkaline – which he believed could better support the body's natural healing processes and overall vitality. For a list of hybrid foods, you can refer to Chapter 3.

Adhering to these principles can help you improve your general health, prevent disease, and create a state of optimal well-being. Dr. Sebi's philosophy continues to inspire and guide those seeking a natural approach to health and wellness.

The Science Behind Alkalinity and Anti-Inflammation

The scientific basis for Dr. Sebi's dietary recommendations digs into the delicate balance of pH levels within the body and its significant impact on general health and wellness. Like we explained in the core principles, the pH scale measures the acidity or alkalinity of a substance, ranging from 0 (highly acidic) to 14 (highly alkaline), with 7 being neutral. In the human body, maintaining a balanced pH is crucial for optimal physiological function. Blood pH, for instance, is tightly regulated within a narrow range, typically between 7.35 and 7.45. Even slight deviations from this range can disrupt essential biological processes. Consuming acidic foods and beverages can disrupt the body's delicate pH balance, leading to a condition known as acidosis. Acidosis occurs when there is an excess of acidity in the body, creating an environment that promotes inflammation, oxidative stress, and the development of various health conditions. Chronic acidosis has been associated with a higher risk of cardiovascular disease, diabetes, arthritis, cancer, and other chronic ailments.

Dr. Sebi's dietary recommendations center on promoting alkalinity within the body to counteract the effects of acidosis and inflammation. Alkaline foods, such as fresh fruits, vegetables, nuts, seeds, and whole grains, play a crucial role in neutralizing acidity and supporting cellular health. These foods are not only low in acidity but are also rich in essential nutrients, antioxidants, vitamins, and minerals, which bolster the body's natural detoxification processes and strengthen the immune system. The inclusion of alkaline foods also supports cellular regeneration, tissue repair, and the body's ability to combat oxidative stress. Additionally, you may experience increased energy levels, improved digestion, enhanced mental clarity, and a reduced risk of chronic diseases such as obesity, type 2 diabetes, and cardiovascular ailments.

In a word, the science behind alkalinity and anti-inflammation underscores the intricate interplay between pH balance, nutrition, and overall health. You can promote optimal cellular function, reduce inflammation, and begin on a revolutionary path towards holistic health and vitality by adhering to nature's principals and eating an alkaline and anti-inflammatory diet.

How Dr. Sebi's Diet Differs from Traditional Healthy Diets?

Dr. Sebi's diet differs significantly from traditional "healthy" diets in several key aspects. Unlike conventional diets, which often include a balance of fruits, vegetables, lean meats, dairy, and whole grains, Dr. Sebi's diet strictly eliminates all animal products, processed foods, and hybrid foods, advocating for a fully vegan and natural eating plan.

One of the most notable differences is Dr. Sebi's focus on maintaining an alkaline internal environment. Traditional healthy diets, such as the Mediterranean or DASH diets, focus on nutrient balance and reducing unhealthy fats, sugars, and salts. In contrast, Dr. Sebi's diet categorizes foods based on their potential to produce alkaline or acidic effects in the body. This diet promotes foods that are believed to help maintain a slightly alkaline pH level, which Dr. Sebi claimed could prevent disease and promote healing by reducing mucus buildup, which he believed to be the root cause of many ailments.

Another distinction lies in the types of foods recommended. Dr. Sebi's nutritional guide emphasizes consuming specific fruits, vegetables, nuts, seeds, and grains that are considered "electric" and non-hybridized, meaning they are in their natural state and not genetically modified or crossbred. This includes items like amaranth, quinoa, spelt, and teff, as well as a variety of less commonly known fruits and vegetables. Traditional healthy diets might include a wider variety of plant-based foods, including those that are genetically modified or hybridized, as long as they provide essential nutrients and vitamins.

The diet also incorporates a significant emphasis on herbal remedies. Dr. Sebi promoted the use of various herbs to cleanse and detoxify the body, support organ function, and enhance overall well-being. This holistic approach is less common in traditional diets, which may recommend supplements but do not typically integrate specific herbal protocols as a core component.

Additionally, Dr. Sebi's diet is deeply rooted in the philosophy of holistic health and natural healing. It encourages lifestyle changes beyond diet, such as fasting, proper hydration with natural spring water, and avoidance of non-natural substances. Traditional healthy diets often focus more on balanced nutrition and exercise, without the broader lifestyle implications emphasized in Dr. Sebi's teachings.

Overall, while traditional healthy diets aim to provide a balanced intake of nutrients to maintain overall health and prevent chronic diseases, Dr. Sebi's diet advocates for a specific selection of natural, alkaline foods and holistic practices aimed at creating an optimal internal environment for healing and disease prevention. This distinct approach reflects Dr. Sebi's unique perspective on health and wellness, emphasizing natural, plant-based nutrition and holistic care.

Is the Dr. Sebi Diet for You?

The ultimate answer is for you to decide, but since you've picked up this book, it's possible you're dealing with certain life circumstances that are forcing you to look for ways to get better. If you are grappling with chronic health issues such as hypertension, diabetes, or autoimmune diseases, you might seek alternative approaches to complement traditional treatments. Dr. Sebi's diet emphasizes natural, alkaline foods that are believed to reduce inflammation and promote healing. Many followers report improvements in their conditions, feeling more energized and experiencing fewer symptoms. The diet's focus on eliminating processed foods and emphasizing nutrient-rich, plant-based options can potentially lead to better management of chronic diseases.

Another common reason for practitioners is the appeal of nature. You might be inclined toward a more natural and holistic approach to health and wellness. Dr. Sebi's philosophy centers around the idea that natural, plant-based foods are the most beneficial for human health. If you prefer to avoid pharmaceuticals and seek natural remedies for health issues, this diet aligns well with those values. The emphasis on herbal supplements and detoxifying the body can appeal to those who believe in the healing power of nature.

Maybe it's none of the above reasons and you're just interested in fitness. Weight loss and increased energy are common reasons for adopting new diets. Dr. Sebi's diet, being rich in fruits, vegetables, nuts, seeds, and grains, is naturally low in calories and high in fiber, which can promote weight loss. The elimination of processed foods and sugars can also lead to increased energy levels. If you feel sluggish or struggle with weight management, this diet's focus on whole, unprocessed foods might offer the benefits you seek.

Some people opt for the alkaline path on ethical and environmental considerations. Dr. Sebi's diet is fully plant-based, aligning with vegan and vegetarian principles that oppose animal cruelty and support sustainable eating practices. If you are concerned about the environmental impact of your food choices, adopting this diet can help reduce your carbon footprint and support more sustainable agricultural practices.

Perhaps you stumbled across the "magic" diet that cures chronic diseases. You might be inspired by personal testimonials and success stories from individuals who have experienced positive changes after adopting Dr. Sebi's diet. Stories of people reversing chronic illnesses, achieving significant weight loss, and gaining a renewed sense of health and vitality can be very motivating. These anecdotal successes can offer hope and a sense of community as you embark on your health journey. For some, the diet resonates on a cultural or spiritual level. Dr. Sebi's philosophy includes elements of African traditional medicine and holistic health practices. If these aspects align with your cultural background or spiritual beliefs, you might find a deeper connection to the diet beyond its health benefits.

Finally, you might simply be in a place in your life where you are seeking change and renewal. Whether you've struggled with yo-yo dieting, faced health scares, or felt disconnected from your body, adopting Dr. Sebi's diet can represent a fresh start. The structured, disciplined approach can provide a sense of control and a path to rebuilding your health from the inside out.

If these are your reasons, you're in the right place. This book not only offers a variety of recipes but also includes a detailed 28-day plan to help you detox your body and restore its natural balance. By following this structured program, you'll gradually eliminate harmful substances and replace them with nourishing, alkaline foods. Each day is carefully planned to ensure a smooth transition, providing meals and tips that support your body's detoxification process. At the end of the 28 days, you'll feel rejuvenated, healthier, and more in tune with your body's natural rhythms.

CHAPTER 2

The Importance of Alkaline and Anti-Inflammatory Diets

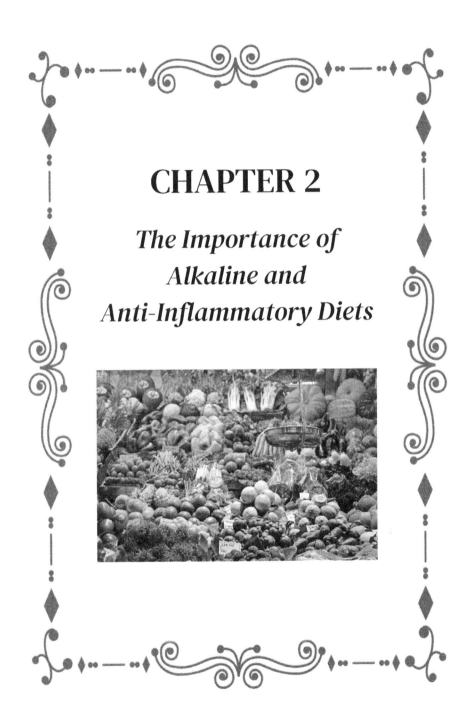

U nderstanding the importance of alkaline and anti-inflammatory diets is crucial for achieving optimal health and well-being. This chapter delves into the science behind these dietary approaches, exploring how they can help reduce chronic inflammation, balance the body's pH levels, and prevent various health issues. By adopting an alkaline and anti-inflammatory diet, you can enhance your body's natural healing processes, boost your immune system, and improve overall vitality. This chapter will provide you with the knowledge and tools needed to make informed dietary choices that support long-term health and wellness.

Benefits of an Alkaline Diet

An alkaline diet, central to Dr. Sebi's teachings, is designed to maintain a balanced pH level in the body, promoting overall health and vitality. This dietary approach emphasizes the consumption of natural, plant-based foods that help keep the body's pH level slightly alkaline, which is crucial for optimal health.

1. Improved Cellular Function

Cells thrive in a slightly alkaline environment, where they can carry out essential processes efficiently. An alkaline pH facilitates optimal cellular metabolism, allowing cells to absorb nutrients effectively and eliminate waste products efficiently. In contrast, an acidic environment disrupts these processes, impairing cellular function and compromising overall health.

One of the key benefits of an alkaline diet is its ability to promote cellular energy production. Within cells, energy is generated through a process called cellular respiration, which occurs most efficiently in an alkaline environment. When the body becomes too acidic due to factors such as diet, stress, or environmental toxins, cellular respiration can be impaired, leading to decreased energy production and feelings of fatigue and lethargy.

In addition to energy production, maintaining an alkaline cellular environment supports optimal immune function. The immune system relies on healthy, properly functioning cells to mount an effective response against pathogens and foreign invaders. In an acidic environment, immune cells may become less effective at carrying out their protective functions, leaving the body more vulnerable to infections and illness. By contrast, an alkaline environment supports the proper functioning of immune cells, helping to enhance immune surveillance and response.

Furthermore, an alkaline cellular environment promotes efficient detoxification. Cells constantly encounter toxins and metabolic waste products that must be eliminated to maintain health. In an alkaline environment, cells can more effectively neutralize and eliminate these toxins, reducing the burden on the body's detoxification organs, such as the liver and kidneys. This supports overall detoxification processes and helps prevent the accumulation of harmful substances that can contribute to chronic disease.

Beyond these direct effects on cellular function, an alkaline diet also provides cells with essential nutrients needed for optimal health and vitality. These nutrients play critical roles in maintaining cellular integrity, regulating gene expression, and protecting cells from oxidative damage and inflammation.

2. Enhanced Detoxification

Alkaline foods, abundant in leafy greens, fruits, nuts, and seeds, are replete with antioxidants and phytonutrients crucial for neutralizing free radicals within the body. These free radicals, when left unmanaged, induce oxidative stress, paving the way for cellular damage and chronic inflammation. Including alkaline-rich foods in your diet can enhance your body's natural detoxification mechanisms, aiding in the elimination of toxins and lowering the risk of chronic diseases. This detoxification process not only aids in disease prevention but also revitalizes overall well-being and elevates energy levels, fostering a sense of vitality and health.

3. Better Bone Health

When the body becomes overly acidic, it may resort to leaching calcium and other essential minerals from the bones to counteract this acidity. Over time, this process can weaken the bones, leading to conditions like osteoporosis and increasing the risk of fractures. However, if you adopt an alkaline diet, you can assist in maintaining a stable pH balance in your body, which decreases the demand for calcium release from the bones as a buffer. Preserving bone density and strength is crucial for averting bone disorders and maintaining skeletal health, especially as you grow older. By giving priority to alkaline foods abundant in nutrients that bolster bone health, you can strengthen your skeletal framework and lower the risk of fractures and osteoporosis, ultimately fostering long-term bone health and vitality.

4. Increased Energy Levels and Mental Clarity

Unlike acidic foods, which might make you feel lethargic and mentally foggy, alkaline foods provide sustained energy and sharper cognitive function. This improvement in vitality and mental acuity stems from several factors inherent to alkaline nutrition. Firstly, alkaline foods tend to optimize metabolic processes, ensuring that the body efficiently converts nutrients into usable energy. Additionally, an alkaline environment supports better oxygenation of tissues, which is essential for cellular energy production and overall vitality.

Moreover, alkaline foods are typically rich in essential nutrients, including vitamins, minerals, antioxidants, and phytonutrients. These nutrients play vital roles in various physiological processes, from supporting cellular function to enhancing brain health. For instance, vitamins like B-complex vitamins and vitamin C are crucial for energy metabolism and neurotransmitter synthesis, contributing to increased alertness and mental clarity.

Furthermore, the abundance of antioxidants in alkaline foods helps protect against oxidative stress, which can impair cognitive function and contribute to feelings of fatigue. By neutralizing free radicals and reducing inflammation, antioxidants support optimal brain health and function, allowing for improved focus, concentration, and cognitive performance.

The nutrient density and alkalizing properties of an alkaline diet translates into sustained energy levels, enhanced mental clarity, and better overall performance in both physical and cognitive tasks.

5. Weight Management

Many alkaline foods are naturally low in calories while being high in fiber. Incorporating a mix of these foods into your diet keeps you feeling full for longer, curbing overeating and fostering a feeling of satisfaction after meals. Moreover, the high fiber content of alkaline foods plays a crucial role in weight management. Fiber adds bulk to the diet, which not only contributes to feelings of fullness but also slows down the digestion and absorption of nutrients. This slower digestion process helps regulate blood sugar levels, preventing spikes that can lead to overeating and weight gain. Additionally, fiber supports digestive health by promoting regular bowel movements and preventing constipation, which can contribute to weight retention.

Furthermore, an alkaline diet is associated with a reduction in inflammation and improvement in insulin sensitivity. Chronic inflammation and insulin resistance are key contributors to obesity and metabolic disorders like type 2 diabetes. Eating foods that help lower inflammation and support proper insulin function can minimize these risk factors and enhance metabolic health. This can lead to more efficient energy use, less fat storage, and an overall improvement in body composition.

The combination of reduced calorie intake, improved satiety, and enhanced metabolic function makes an alkaline diet a valuable tool for achieving and maintaining a healthy weight.

6. Reduced Inflammation

Chronic inflammation is a recognized contributor to various health issues, spanning from cardiovascular disease and arthritis to autoimmune disorders. Alkaline-rich foods, abundant in antioxidants, vitamins, and minerals, are pivotal in modulating the body's inflammatory responses. By neutralizing harmful free radicals and suppressing inflammatory pathways, these nutrient-dense foods work to alleviate inflammation at the cellular level. Transitioning towards a diet centered on alkaline options creates an internal environment less conducive to chronic inflammation. This dietary shift not only addresses inflammation symptoms but also targets underlying factors contributing to its onset.

Adopting an alkaline diet offers a comprehensive approach to inflammation reduction and the promotion of long-term health and vigor You can reduce the risk of chronic inflammatory disorders and create an internal environment that supports normal cellular function by consuming fewer acidic foods and more alkaline-rich foods.

7. Enhanced Cardiovascular Health

An alkaline diet offers notable benefits for cardiovascular health. One of the primary ways is by reducing inflammation. Chronic inflammation is a known risk factor for heart disease, as it can damage blood vessels and contribute to the formation of arterial plaque. Alkaline foods, rich in antioxidants and phytonutrients, help combat inflammation throughout the body, including the cardiovascular system.

Additionally, an alkaline diet can positively influence cholesterol levels, another critical aspect of cardiovascular health. High levels of LDL cholesterol, often referred to as "bad" cholesterol, can lead to the buildup of plaque in the arteries, increasing the risk of heart attack and stroke. Alkaline foods, particularly those high in soluble fiber, help lower LDL cholesterol levels by binding to cholesterol molecules and promoting their excretion from the body. You can lower your blood pressure and safeguard your heart by consuming a diet high in fiber-rich foods including fruits, vegetables, and whole grains.

8. Longevity and Vitality

An alkaline diet offers more than just short-term health benefits; it contributes to longevity and vitality over the long term. An alkaline diet can help you stay healthy as you get older by lowering the chances of developing chronic conditions like heart disease, diabetes, and cancer. The high nutrient density of alkaline foods provides the body with essential vitamins, minerals, and antioxidants, supporting optimal bodily functions and overall well-being. Additionally, the sustained energy levels provided by alkaline foods contribute to vitality and a higher quality of life. Adopting an alkaline diet can support your body's natural healing processes and lead to a longer, healthier life filled with vitality and well-being.

The benefits of an alkaline diet are vast and varied, encompassing improved cellular function, enhanced detoxification, better bone health, increased energy and mental clarity, effective weight management, reduced inflammation, improved immune function, enhanced digestive health, better skin health, and enhanced cardiovascular health. In line with Dr. Sebi's holistic approach to wellbeing, you can lay the groundwork for long-lasting health and vigour by concentrating on a diet high in natural, plant-based foods.

How Anti-Inflammatory Foods Combat Illness

Chronic inflammation, often referred to as "silent inflammation," is a pervasive yet insidious process that underlies the pathogenesis of various chronic diseases. Unlike acute inflammation, which is the body's rapid and localized response to injury or infection, chronic inflammation persists over an extended period, often silently smoldering within tissues and organs. This persistent low-grade inflammation can gradually inflict damage on cellular structures, disrupt physiological processes, and contribute to the development and progression of debilitating health conditions. The detrimental effects of chronic inflammation extend across multiple organ systems and are implicated in a diverse array of diseases. Cardiovascular diseases, including atherosclerosis, hypertension, and coronary artery disease, are closely linked to chronic inflammation. Inflammatory processes within the arterial walls promote the accumulation of plaque, narrowing blood vessels and increasing the risk of heart attacks and strokes. Similarly, chronic inflammation plays a pivotal role in the pathogenesis of metabolic disorders such as type 2 diabetes and obesity. Inflammation disrupts insulin signaling pathways, leading to insulin resistance and dysregulated glucose metabolism. Persistent low-grade inflammation in adipose tissue contributes to the secretion of pro-inflammatory cytokines and adipokines, fostering a state of chronic metabolic dysfunction.

Cancer, characterized by uncontrolled cellular proliferation and tumor growth, is also intricately intertwined with chronic inflammation. Inflammatory mediators in the tumor microenvironment promote tumor initiation, progression, and metastasis by modulating immune responses, angiogenesis, and DNA damage repair mechanisms. Chronic inflammation creates a tumor-promoting milieu that fuels oncogenic processes and facilitates tumor evasion of immune surveillance. Neurodegenerative diseases like Alzheimer's disease and Parkinson's disease are increasingly recognized as inflammatory conditions with neuroinflammation playing a central role in disease progression. Chronic activation of microglia, the resident immune cells of the central nervous system, contributes to neuronal damage, synaptic loss, and cognitive decline observed in these.

Furthermore, autoimmune disorders, characterized by aberrant immune responses targeting self-antigens, are fueled by chronic inflammation. Dysregulated immune responses lead to tissue damage and dysfunction in organs and systems targeted by autoimmune attacks. Inflammatory cytokines and chemokines orchestrate the inflammatory cascade, perpetuating autoimmune pathology and contributing to disease flares.

With this, we can see how damaging inflammation can be. To counteract these effects, Dr. Sebi's philosophy stresses anti-inflammatory foods. One of the pivotal roles of anti-inflammatory foods lies in their profound ability to counteract oxidative stress, a process implicated in the development and progression of chronic diseases. Oxidative stress ensues when there's an imbalance between the production of free radicals—highly reactive molecules containing unpaired electrons—and the body's antioxidant defenses. These free radicals, in their quest to stabilize themselves, can indiscriminately attack cellular components such as DNA, proteins, and lipids, initiating a cascade of molecular damage and inflammatory responses. Here, anti-inflammatory foods emerge as potent allies in the fight against oxidative stress. These foods are densely packed with a plethora of antioxidants, including vitamins C and E, beta-carotene, selenium, and numerous phytochemicals, all of which act as molecular scavengers, intercepting and neutralizing free radicals before they wreak havoc on cellular structures. By effectively quenching these harmful radicals, anti-inflammatory foods serve as guardians of cellular integrity, shielding vital biomolecules from oxidative damage and preventing the propagation of inflammatory cascades.

Omega-3 fatty acids, a class of polyunsaturated fats hailed for their myriad health benefits, play a particularly noteworthy role in dampening inflammation and mitigating oxidative stress. Abundant in certain plant-based sources such as flaxseeds, chia seeds, hemp seeds, and walnuts, these fatty acids serve as precursors to specialized pro-resolving mediators (SPMs)—bioactive lipid-derived molecules instrumental in orchestrating the resolution of inflammation. SPMs exert their anti-inflammatory prowess by modulating inflammatory signaling pathways, promoting the clearance of inflammatory debris, and facilitating tissue repair and regeneration. You can take advantage of the strong anti-inflammatory qualities of omega-3 fatty acids by adding these items to their diet and strengthening their body's resistance to disorders linked to chronic inflammation.

The fiber content of anti-inflammatory foods also plays an indispensable role in nurturing gut health and orchestrating inflammation modulation. Dietary fiber, a complex carbohydrate found abundantly in plant-based foods, serves as a prebiotic—a substance that fuels the growth and activity of beneficial gut bacteria. Fibre supports a varied and robust gut microbiome makeup, which is essential for immunological control and inflammatory balance, by feeding these symbiotic microorganisms. And it's not just about immune health—fiber-rich foods also help regulate your blood sugar levels. They slow down the absorption of sugar from your gut, preventing sudden spikes in blood sugar that can trigger inflammation. This is especially important for people with insulin resistance or type 2 diabetes, as it helps reduce the inflammation caused by unstable blood sugar levels.

Phytochemicals, bioactive compounds inherent to plants, wield remarkable anti-inflammatory properties that contribute to overall health and wellness. Polyphenols, such as those found in herbal teas and berries, exhibit potent antioxidant and anti-inflammatory effects, scavenging free radicals and dampening inflammatory signaling pathways within the body.

Utilize the synergistic action of fiber, phytochemicals, and other bioactive constituents found in anti-inflammatory foods. This will help you nurture a nourishing internal environment that supports optimal health and well-being, establishing a foundation for sustained vitality and resilience against inflammatory challenges.

Preventing Disease Through Diet

Plant-based foods, such as fruits, vegetables, nuts, seeds, and whole grains, are rich sources of vitamins, minerals, antioxidants, and phytonutrients that possess potent anti-inflammatory properties. These bioactive compounds neutralize harmful free radicals, dampen inflammatory signaling, and support the body's natural defense mechanisms against inflammation-related damage. Including a wide variety of colorful fruits and vegetables in your diet enables you to benefit from the combined effects of these phytonutrients, promoting optimal health and aiding in disease prevention. Antioxidants abundant in plant foods play a crucial role in disease prevention by protecting cells from oxidative damage. By neutralizing free radicals, antioxidants preserve cellular integrity and support overall health.

Maintaining a healthy weight is essential for disease prevention, as obesity is a significant risk factor for various metabolic disorders and chronic conditions. A plant-based diet, naturally lower in calorie density and higher in fiber content, can facilitate weight management and promote satiety, leading to reduced calorie intake and improved metabolic health. Dietary fiber not only promotes feelings of fullness but also supports digestive health and regulates blood sugar levels, contributing further to weight control and disease prevention. Stable blood sugar levels, achieved by prioritizing whole, unprocessed foods with a low glycemic index, reduce the risk of developing diabetes and metabolic disorders.

Heart health is another critical area influenced by dietary choices. Consuming foods rich in healthy fats, such as omega-3 fatty acids found in flaxseeds, chia seeds, and walnuts, can lower cholesterol levels, reduce blood pressure, and prevent the development of atherosclerosis. These fats support cardiovascular function by reducing inflammation, improving blood vessel function, and lowering the risk of blood clot formation. Additionally, antioxidant-rich foods like berries and leafy greens help protect against oxidative stress and inflammation, key drivers of heart disease.

Gut health is vital for overall well-being and disease prevention. A diet rich in fiber, prebiotics, and probiotics supports a healthy gut microbiome, which plays a crucial role in immune function, nutrient absorption, and inflammation regulation. Fiber acts as a prebiotic, nourishing beneficial gut bacteria and promoting microbial diversity, which is associated with improved immune function and reduced inflammation. Probiotic-rich foods like yogurt and kimchi further enhance gut health and support immune function. Embracing a plant-based diet not only provides essential nutrients and bioactive compounds but also promotes a healthy gut, contributing to overall health and resilience against diseases.

Preventing cancer through diet is a foundational aspect of Dr. Sebi's holistic health philosophy. Embrace a plant-based, anti-inflammatory diet rich in phytochemicals, antioxidants, fiber, and other protective nutrients to proactively reduce your risk of developing cancer and support your body's natural defense mechanisms against this devastating disease. This proactive approach to health and wellness aligns with the body's innate healing abilities and promotes long-term vitality and well-being.

CHAPTER 3

Essentials of the Alkaline Diet

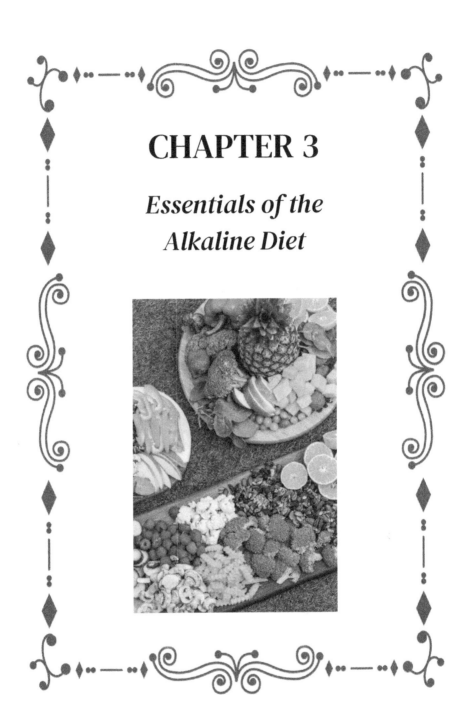

The alkaline diet, hailed for its potential health benefits and emphasis on whole, nutrient-dense foods, has garnered significant attention in recent years. Rooted in the concept of maintaining a balanced pH level in the body, this dietary approach aims to optimize health and vitality by promoting alkaline-forming foods while minimizing acidic choices. In this chapter, we look at the essentials of an alkaline diet.

Key Components of an Alkaline Diet

The primary components of the alkaline diet include fresh fruits, vegetables, nuts, seeds, and whole grains. These foods are naturally abundant in essential vitamins, minerals, antioxidants, and phytonutrients, all of which play crucial roles in supporting overall well-being.

Fresh Fruits and Vegetables

Foundational elements of the alkaline diet, fresh fruits, and vegetables form the cornerstone of this nutritional approach due to their highly alkaline-forming nature. These plant-based foods are rich sources of essential vitamins, minerals, antioxidants, and phytochemicals, all of which play crucial roles in supporting overall well-being.

Recommended options include:

- leafy greens like kale,
- berries like strawberries, blueberries, and raspberries,
- citrus fruits like lemons, oranges, and grapefruits,
- and root vegetables like burdock root, dandelion root, and sarsaparilla root.

These alkaline-forming foods help create a favorable pH balance within the body, supporting cellular function and detoxification processes.

Nuts and Seeds

Nuts and seeds play a pivotal role in the alkaline diet, offering valuable nutrients such as fatty acids, protein, and minerals. While some varieties may be more acidic (such as peanuts), others like walnuts, hemp seeds, and raw sesame seeds are alkaline-forming and provide numerous health benefits. Walnuts, for example, are rich in omega-3 fatty acids, magnesium, and healthy fats, while hemp seeds are a great source of protein and essential fatty acids. These nutritious snacks can be seamlessly integrated into meals or enjoyed as standalone snacks, providing sustained energy levels and a sense of satiety. Approved nuts and seeds in Dr. Sebi's diet include:

- walnuts,
- hemp seeds,
- raw sesame seeds, and
- Brazil nuts.

Whole Grains

Whole grains are favored over refined grains in the alkaline diet due to their lower acidity and higher nutrient content. Options such as:

- quinoa,
- amaranth,
- spelt,
- teff,
- and wild rice

are alkaline-forming and provide complex carbohydrates, fiber, vitamins, and minerals. These whole grains contribute to stabilizing blood sugar levels, supporting digestive health, and sustaining energy levels throughout the day. Unlike refined grains, which are stripped of their bran and germ during processing, whole grains retain their fiber content, promoting satiety and digestive regularity.

Understanding pH and Your Health

Maintaining pH balance in the body is essential for optimal health and proper physiological function. The body's pH, particularly the blood, is kept within a narrow range of 7.35 to 7.45, which is slightly alkaline. This balance is crucial for enzyme function, metabolic processes, and cellular activities. Enzymes, which catalyze biochemical reactions, work best at specific pH levels, and deviations can impair their activity, leading to metabolic disruptions. Additionally, cellular functions such as nutrient transport and waste removal depend on maintaining an optimal pH level.

Different parts of the digestive system require varying pH levels; for instance, the stomach needs to be highly acidic for digestion, while the small intestine requires a more alkaline environment for nutrient absorption. Proper pH balance also supports immune function and bone health. Chronic acidity can lead to bone demineralization as the body uses minerals like calcium to buffer excess acid, potentially resulting in weakened bones and osteoporosis. To maintain pH balance, a diet rich in fruits, vegetables, and whole grains while limiting processed foods and refined sugars is recommended.

Health Considerations of Dr. Sebi's Diet

While Dr. Sebi's diet is praised for its emphasis on natural, plant-based foods, there are several health risks and concerns associated with following it strictly. Here are some potential health risks you should consider before start your first diet:

1. **Nutritional Deficiencies**

   One of the primary concerns with Dr. Sebi's diet is the potential for nutritional deficiencies. The diet eliminates many food groups, including animal products, dairy, and certain grains, which are primary sources of essential nutrients such as protein, calcium, iron, vitamin B12, and omega-3 fatty acids. Without careful planning, individuals might struggle to obtain sufficient amounts of these nutrients, leading to deficiencies that can cause issues such as anemia, weakened bones, and impaired immune function.

2. **Limited Protein Sources**

   The diet's restriction of animal products significantly reduces the available sources of complete proteins, which contain all essential amino acids. While some plant-based foods do provide protein, they may not offer a complete amino acid profile unless combined properly. This can be particularly challenging for individuals with higher protein needs, such as athletes, growing children, or those recovering from illness or surgery.

3. **Potential for Unbalanced Diet**

   Dr. Sebi's diet emphasizes specific foods and herbs, which might lead to an unbalanced diet if not carefully managed. For example, focusing heavily on certain fruits and vegetables while neglecting others can result in an unbalanced intake of nutrients. Over-reliance on a limited variety of foods can also make it challenging to maintain a nutritionally adequate diet over the long term.

4. **Risk of Overdoing Detoxification**

   The diet promotes detoxification practices, including fasting and the use of certain herbs. While detoxing can have benefits, excessive or improper detoxification can lead to dehydration, electrolyte imbalances, and nutrient depletion. Fasting for extended periods without medical supervision can also be dangerous, particularly for individuals with underlying health conditions.

5. **Scientific Validation and Safety Concerns**

   The principles of Dr. Sebi's diet, including the strict avoidance of hybrid foods and the emphasis on an alkaline diet, lack substantial scientific validation. While eating a diet rich in fruits and vegetables is widely recognized as healthy, the specific claims about alkalinity and hybrid foods are not well-supported by scientific evidence. This lack of validation means that some of the diet's recommendations may not be as beneficial as claimed, and could potentially be harmful.

6. **Social and Practical Challenges**

   Strict adherence to Dr. Sebi's diet can pose social and practical challenges. The diet's limitations can make it difficult to eat out, attend social gatherings, or find suitable food options in some regions. This can lead to social isolation or stress, which can negatively impact mental health and overall well-being.

7. **Potential for Misuse or Misinterpretation**

   As with any diet, there is a risk that individuals may misuse or misinterpret the guidelines. This can lead to overly restrictive eating patterns, which may result in disordered eating behaviors. Without proper guidance, individuals might also fail to recognize when adjustments or supplementation are necessary to meet their nutritional needs.

In summary, while Dr. Sebi's diet offers potential benefits through its focus on natural, plant-based foods, it also carries significant health risks if not followed carefully. It's essential for individuals considering this diet to seek professional medical advice and ensure they are meeting all their nutritional needs. Balancing the diet with a variety of nutrient-dense foods and possibly incorporating supplements can help mitigate some of these risks.

Now that we've given you the disclaimer, we can start exploring the food groups allowed and prohibited in this diet.

Foods to Embrace and Avoid

Approved Foods

Vegetables

- Amaranth Greens
- Avocado
- Bell Peppers
- Chayote
- Cucumber
- Dandelion Greens
- Garbanzo Beans (Chickpeas)
- Izote (Cactus Flower)
- Kale
- Lettuce (Except Iceberg)
- Mushrooms (Except Shitake)
- Nopales (Mexican Cactus)
- Okra
- Olives
- Onions
- Purslane (Verdolaga)
- Sea Vegetables (Wakame, Dulse, Arame, Hijiki, Nori, Sea Moss)
- Squash (Except Pumpkin)
- Tomatoes (Cherry and Plum Only)
- Turnip Greens
- Watercress
- Wild Arugula
- Zucchini

Fruits

- Apples
- Bananas (Burro/Mid-Size)
- Berries (All Varieties Except Cranberries)
- Cantaloupe
- Cherries
- Currants
- Dates
- Figs
- Grapes (Seeded)
- Limes (Key Limes Preferred)
- Mango
- Melons (Seeded)
- Oranges (Seville/Sour)
- Papayas
- Peaches
- Pears
- Plums
- Prickly Pear (Cactus Fruit)
- Prunes
- Raisins (Seeded)
- Soft Jelly Coconut (Coconut Jelly)
- Soursop

Grains

- Amaranth
- Fonio
- Kamut
- Quinoa
- Rye
- Spelt
- Teff
- Wild Rice

Nuts and Seeds

- Brazil Nuts
- Hemp Seeds
- Raw Sesame Seeds
- Walnuts

Oils

- Olive Oil (Do Not Cook)
- Coconut Oil (Do Not Cook)
- Grapeseed Oil
- Hempseed Oil
- Avocado Oil

Spices and Seasonings

- Basil
- Bay Leaf
- Cloves
- Dill
- Oregano
- Onion Powder
- Pure Sea Salt

- Sage
- Savory
- Sweet Basil
- Tarragon
- Thyme

Herbal Teas

- Burdock
- Chamomile
- Elderberry
- Fennel
- Ginger
- Red Raspberry
- Cuachalalate
- Flor de Manita
- Gordo Lobo
- Muicle

Foods to Avoid

Animal Products

- Meat
- Poultry
- Fish
- Eggs
- Dairy
- Honey

Processed Meats

- Bacon
- Hotdogs

Processed Foods

- White Flour
- White Sugar
- Artificial Sweeteners
- Packaged Foods

Processed Flours and Grains

- White Flour
- Bleached Flour
- Self-Rising Flour
- Enriched Flour
- White Rice
- White Pasta
- Crackers
- Cereal

Refined Oils

- Soybean Oil
- Canola Oil
- Corn Oil

Acidic Beverages

- Coffee
- Tea
- Alcohol

Junk Food

- Fast Food
- Chips
- Candy
- Cake
- Cookies
- Pies

Hybrid Foods

- **Hybrid Fruits**
  o Seedless Grapes
  o Seedless Watermelons
  o Cavendish Bananas
- **Hybrid Vegetables**
  o Broccoli
  o Cauliflower
  o Carrots
  o Corn
  o Beets
- **Hybrid Spices and Herbs**
  o Aloe
  o Mint
  o Turmeric
- **Hybrid Lemons (supermarket variety)**

Microwaved Meals

- Any Microwaved Food

Canned Foods

- Canned Fruits
- Canned Vegetables
- High-Sodium Additives

Artificial Ingredients

- MSG
- Artificial Colors
- Artificial Flavors

Artificial Sweeteners

- Equal
- Splenda
- NutraSweet
- Sweet'N Low

Fast Foods

- Ready-Made Meals
- Frozen Dinners
- Takeaways

Chemically-Altered Foods

- Margarine
- Shortening
- Trans Fats
- Vegetable Oils
- Aspartame
- BHA
- BHT
- TBHQ

Diet and Processed Low-Fat Products

- Diet Soda
- Low-Fat Cookies
- Reduced Fat Peanut Butter

Packaged Drinks

- Soft Drinks
- Sports Drinks
- Energy Drinks
- Fruit Juices
- Soda Water
- Sparkling Water

GMO Foods

- Corn
- Commercially Processed Flours
- Corn Meal
- Soybeans
- Canola Oil

Yeast Products

- Breads
- Cakes
- Buns

Pesticide-Ridden Foods

- Non-Organic Fruits and Vegetables
- Non-Organic Meat, Poultry, Dairy

Preservatives

- BHA
- BHT
- TBHQ
- Sodium Nitrate
- Sodium Benzoate

Other Manmade Products

- Growth Hormones
- rBGH/rBST
- Antibiotics
- Steroids
- Irradiated Food

CHAPTER 4

Building Blocks of the Anti-Inflammatory Diet

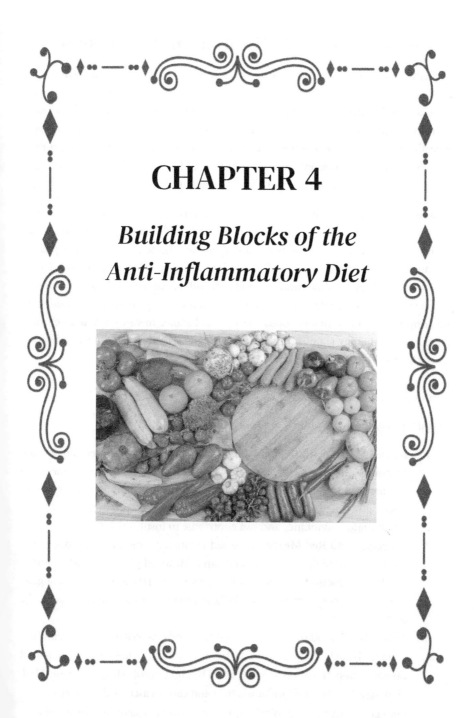

Inflammatory vs. Anti-Inflammatory Foods

Inflammatory foods encompass those dietary components that possess the potential to instigate or exacerbate inflammation processes within the body, consequently contributing to the initiation or progression of chronic diseases such as heart disease, diabetes, arthritis, and certain cancers. These dietary culprits typically exhibit high concentrations of refined sugars, unhealthy fats, and artificial additives, all of which not only have the capacity to induce oxidative stress but also disrupt the body's innate mechanisms for managing inflammatory responses.

Among the roster of common inflammatory foods are processed snacks, sugary beverages, fried delicacies, red meat, refined grains, and items containing trans fats (their exact damaging potential is explained below). These dietary choices possess the capacity to disrupt the delicate balance between pro-inflammatory cytokines—molecules that trigger inflammation—and anti-inflammatory cytokines, which play a crucial role in regulating the body's inflammatory reactions. Consistent consumption of inflammatory foods can tip this balance towards a state of chronic inflammation, thereby significantly heightening the risk of developing a wide array of health ailments.

Common Inflammatory Foods

Several types of foods are known to promote inflammation:

1. **Refined Carbohydrates and Sugars**: Foods high in refined sugars and carbohydrates, such as white bread, pastries, sodas, and other sugar-laden products, can spike blood sugar levels and trigger inflammatory responses. High glycemic index foods lead to increased production of pro-inflammatory cytokines and can contribute to insulin resistance.
2. **Processed and Red Meats**: Processed meats (e.g., sausages, hot dogs) and red meats are high in saturated fats and advanced glycation end products (AGEs), compounds that form when proteins or fats combine with sugars. These substances can promote inflammation and oxidative stress in the body.
3. **Trans Fats**: Found in many fried and fast foods, as well as in margarine and certain baked goods, trans fats are strongly linked to increased inflammation. They raise levels of LDL cholesterol while lowering HDL cholesterol, promoting inflammation and cardiovascular disease risk.
4. **Omega-6 Fatty Acids**: While some omega-6 fatty acids are necessary for health, excessive intake, especially from processed vegetable oils (e.g., corn,

soybean, and sunflower oils), can promote inflammatory pathways. An imbalance between omega-6 and omega-3 fatty acids is a common issue.

5. **Alcohol**: Excessive alcohol consumption can lead to a variety of health problems, including inflammation of the liver and increased production of inflammatory markers throughout the body. Chronic alcohol use is associated with systemic inflammation and increased risk of diseases like liver cirrhosis and pancreatitis.

6. **Gluten and Casein**: For individuals with sensitivities or allergies, such as those with celiac disease or gluten intolerance, gluten (a protein found in wheat, barley, and rye) and casein (a protein in dairy) can trigger significant inflammatory responses.

Biological Mechanisms

The consumption of inflammatory foods affects the body through several biological mechanisms:

*   **Oxidative Stress**: Many inflammatory foods contribute to the production of free radicals, which can damage cells and tissues through oxidative stress. This oxidative damage can trigger inflammatory pathways and contribute to the development of chronic diseases.

*   **Cytokine Production**: Certain foods can increase the production of pro-inflammatory cytokines, which are signaling proteins that regulate inflammation and immune responses. Chronic elevation of these cytokines can lead to systemic inflammation.

*   **Gut Health**: Inflammatory foods can disrupt the balance of the gut microbiome, leading to dysbiosis. An unhealthy gut microbiome can increase intestinal permeability, allowing inflammatory substances to enter the bloodstream and trigger widespread inflammation.

*   **Insulin Resistance**: Foods high in refined sugars and carbohydrates can cause spikes in blood sugar levels, leading to insulin resistance. Insulin resistance is closely linked to chronic inflammation and metabolic syndrome, a cluster of conditions that increase the risk of heart disease, stroke, and diabetes.

On the opposite end of the spectrum, we've study extensively how anti-inflammatory foods serve as allies in combating inflammation within the body while simultaneously promoting overall health and well-being. Predominantly sourced from plant-based origins, these foods boast a wealth of antioxidants, vitamins, minerals, and phytonutrients—potent agents renowned for their ability to counteract oxidative stress and neutralize free radicals. Moreover, anti-inflammatory foods are rich in healthy fats, notably omega-3 fatty acids, revered for their capacity to quell inflammation and bolster cardiovascular health.

A plethora of anti-inflammatory foods exists. Collectively, these nutritional powerhouses work in tandem to modulate the body's inflammatory response by impeding pro-inflammatory pathways while simultaneously encouraging the production of anti-inflammatory compounds. Deliberately prioritize the consumption of anti-inflammatory foods while consciously minimizing intake of their inflammatory counterparts to craft a dietary blueprint that fosters a harmonized inflammatory response and paves the path toward optimal health and vitality.

Creating a Balanced Anti-Inflammatory Meal

Creating a balanced anti-inflammatory meal using Dr. Sebi's approved foods is an excellent way to promote overall health and well-being. This guide provides a detailed step-by-step process for selecting, preparing, and cooking a nutritious meal that aligns with Dr. Sebi's dietary guidelines.

Step-by-Step Guide:

1. Select Your Ingredients:

Base: Choose a whole grain like quinoa or wild rice. Quinoa and wild rice are nutrient-dense grains that are high in fiber and protein, providing sustained energy and promoting digestive health. They are alkaline-forming and non-hybrid, aligning with Dr. Sebi's dietary guidelines.

Vegetables: Include a variety of colorful, alkaline-forming vegetables such as zucchini, bell peppers, kale, and cherry tomatoes. These vegetables are rich in vitamins, minerals, and antioxidants, which help reduce inflammation and support overall health. Colorful vegetables also ensure a broad range of phytonutrients.

Healthy Fats: Use avocado oil or extra virgin olive oil for cooking. Healthy fats like those found in avocado and olive oil are essential for nutrient absorption and have anti-inflammatory properties. These oils are also alkaline-forming and align with Dr. Sebi's guidelines.

Seasonings: Incorporate approved seasonings like thyme, oregano, sea salt, and onion powder. Natural seasonings add flavor without introducing harmful additives. They often have their own health benefits, such as antimicrobial properties and support for digestive health.

Protein Source: Add chickpeas (garbanzo beans) for protein. Chickpeas are a great source of plant-based protein and fiber, supporting muscle maintenance and digestive health. They are also alkaline-forming and fit within Dr. Sebi's dietary framework.

2.. Preparation:

Quinoa: Rinse 1 cup of quinoa thoroughly. Cook according to package instructions (usually 2 cups of water to 1 cup of quinoa). Bring to a boil, reduce heat, and simmer until water is absorbed (about 15 minutes). This will remove saponins, which can cause a bitter taste.

Vegetables: Wash and chop your vegetables. Ensuring they are clean and ready for quick cooking, which helps retain their nutritional value. For this recipe, we will use 1 zucchini, 1 bell pepper, a handful of kale, and a cup of cherry tomatoes.

Chickpeas: If organic varieties are not available and you're using canned chickpeas, rinse thoroughly; this removes excess sodium. If using dried chickpeas, soak them overnight and cook until tender, ensuring they are free from preservatives and additives.

3. Cooking (using a sample recipe)

Quinoa and Vegetable Stir-Fry

Ingredients:

- 1 cup quinoa
- 2 cups water
- 1 zucchini, chopped
- 1 bell pepper, chopped
- 1 cup cherry tomatoes, halved
- 1 cup chopped kale

- 1 cup cooked chickpeas
- 2 tablespoons avocado oil
- 1 teaspoon sea salt
- 1 teaspoon onion powder
- 1 teaspoon dried thyme

Instructions:

1. Rinse quinoa thoroughly under cold water. In a medium saucepan, bring 2 cups of water to a boil. Add quinoa, reduce heat to low, cover, and simmer for about 15 minutes or until water is absorbed. Fluff with a fork.
2. In a large skillet, heat avocado oil over medium heat. Add zucchini and bell pepper, sauté for 5-7 minutes.
3. Add kale and cherry tomatoes to the skillet. Sauté for another 3-5 minutes.
4. Season with sea salt, onion powder, and dried thyme.
5. Add cooked quinoa and chickpeas to the skillet. Stir well and cook for an additional 3-5 minutes.
6. Serve warm, optionally garnished with fresh herbs like parsley or cilantro.

By following these steps and focusing on Dr. Sebi-approved foods, you can create a delicious, balanced anti-inflammatory meal that supports overall health and well-being. Feel free to experiment with ingredients that suit your tastes.

CHAPTER 5

The Ultimate 28-Day Detox Plan

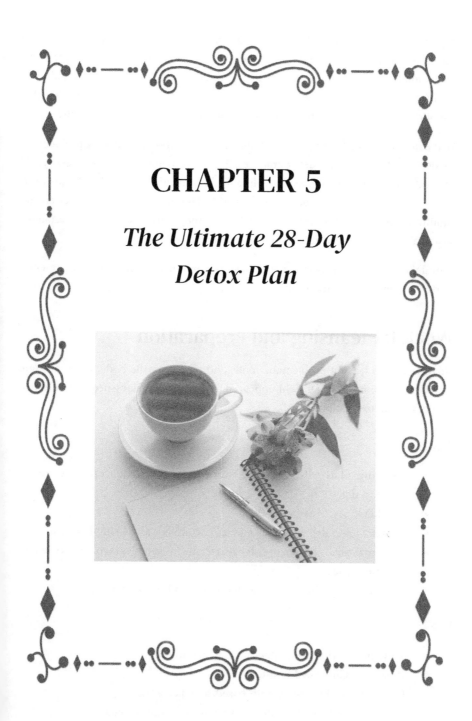

The Ultimate 28-Day Detox Plan is designed to cleanse, rejuvenate, and transform your body and mind. Over the course of four weeks, you'll gradually transition to a nutrient-rich, alkaline diet inspired by Dr. Sebi's principles. This plan is not just about changing what you eat—it's about adopting a holistic lifestyle that supports detoxification, reduces inflammation, and fosters long-term vitality.

In the first week, you'll prepare your body for detoxification by reducing problematic foods and introducing key detox practices. As you move into the second week, you'll integrate more core alkaline foods, feeling the benefits of a cleaner diet. By the third week, you'll deepen the detox with anti-inflammatory recipes, experiencing significant health improvements. Finally, in the fourth week, you'll establish sustainable habits that ensure continued health and well-being.

Throughout this plan, expect to see changes in your energy levels, digestion, mental clarity, and overall physical health.

Week 1: Cleansing and Preparation

Goal: Focus on leaving problematic foods and preparing the body for an alkaline diet. Gradually introduce Dr. Sebi-approved recipes while making necessary lifestyle changes for detoxification.

Day 1:

- **Morning**: Start with a glass of warm water with a squeeze of lemon to kickstart digestion.
- **Breakfast: Sea Moss Smoothie**
- **Lunch**: Light salad with leafy greens, cucumbers, and a simple vinaigrette.
- **Dinner**: Grilled chicken or fish with steamed vegetables (avoid heavy sauces and fried foods).
- **Tip**: Begin reducing the intake of caffeine and sugary beverages.

Day 2:

- **Morning**: Herbal tea (peppermint or chamomile).
- **Breakfast: Chia Seed Pudding**
- **Lunch**: Vegetable soup (broth-based, avoid cream).
- **Dinner**: Baked sweet potatoes with a side of sautéed spinach.
- **Tip**: Increase water intake to at least 8 glasses a day.

Day 3:

- **Morning**: Warm water with apple cider vinegar.
- **Breakfast**: Oatmeal with fresh fruits and nuts.
- **Lunch: Cucumber and Avocado Salad**
- **Dinner**: Lentil soup with a side of steamed broccoli.
- **Tip**: Start incorporating light exercise, such as walking or yoga.

Day 4:

- **Morning**: Fresh vegetable juice (carrots, celery, and apple).
- **Breakfast**: Smoothie bowl with fresh berries and seeds.
- **Lunch**: Grilled vegetables wrap with hummus.
- **Dinner**: Quinoa with roasted vegetables.
- **Tip**: Avoid processed foods and start cooking meals at home.

Day 5:

- **Morning**: Herbal tea (ginger and turmeric).
- **Breakfast: Alkaline Breakfast Smoothie**
- **Lunch**: Large mixed greens salad with avocado, tomatoes, and a light olive oil dressing.
- **Dinner**: Baked salmon with asparagus and a side of brown rice.
- **Tip**: Reduce dairy intake by substituting with plant-based alternatives.

Day 6:

- **Morning**: Lemon water.
- **Breakfast**: Whole grain toast with almond butter and banana slices.
- **Lunch: Butternut Squash and Avocado Toast**
- **Dinner**: Vegetable stir-fry with tofu.
- **Tip**: Start including more raw vegetables in your diet.

Day 7:

- **Morning**: Herbal tea (dandelion root).
- **Breakfast: Amaranth Porridge with Berries**
- **Lunch**: Fresh fruit salad with a variety of seasonal fruits.
- **Dinner**: Brown rice with steamed vegetables and a side of beans.
- **Tip**: Practice mindfulness or meditation to support mental detoxification.

Summary of Week 1:

- **Daily Goals**: Increase water intake, reduce processed foods, and gradually eliminate caffeine, sugar, and dairy.
- **Key Focus**: Start the day with detox drinks like lemon water or herbal teas.
- **Recipes Included**: Sea Moss Smoothie, Chia Seed Pudding, Cucumber and Avocado Salad, Alkaline Breakfast Smoothie, Butternut Squash and Avocado Toast, Amaranth Porridge with Berries.
- **Lifestyle Changes**: Introduce light exercises like walking or yoga, practice mindfulness, and ensure to cook meals at home.

Week 1 sets the foundation for the detox journey by gradually introducing alkaline recipes and making essential lifestyle changes to cleanse the body and prepare it for the following weeks.

Week 2: Integrating Core Alkaline Foods

Goal: Replace most of the diet with Dr. Sebi-approved recipes, while still allowing some flexibility with normal meals. Focus on integrating core alkaline foods and further lifestyle changes to support detoxification.

Day 8:

- **Morning**: Start with warm lemon water.
- **Breakfast: Quinoa Breakfast Bowl with Berries and Nuts**
- **Lunch**: Grilled chicken salad with mixed greens and a light vinaigrette.
- **Dinner: Spelt Pasta with Avocado Pesto**
- **Tip**: Replace one caffeinated beverage with herbal tea.

Day 9:

- **Morning**: Herbal tea (peppermint).
- **Breakfast: Teff Porridge with Fresh Fruit**
- **Lunch**: Quinoa salad with mixed vegetables and a lemon-tahini dressing.
- **Dinner: Chickpea and Wild Rice Stuffed Bell Peppers**
- **Tip**: Begin incorporating more raw foods into meals.

Day 10:

- **Morning**: Warm water with apple cider vinegar.
- **Breakfast: Chia Seed Pudding**
- **Lunch**: Fresh vegetable stir-fry with tofu.
- **Dinner: Amaranth and Vegetable Soup**
- **Tip**: Reduce the intake of refined grains and replace with whole grains.

Day 11:

- **Morning**: Fresh vegetable juice (cucumber, celery, and apple).
- **Breakfast: Alkaline Breakfast Smoothie**
- **Lunch**: Large mixed greens salad with avocado, tomatoes, and a light olive oil dressing.
- **Dinner: Zucchini Noodles with Walnut Pesto**
- **Tip**: Add more leafy greens to daily meals.

Day 12:

- **Morning**: Herbal tea (ginger and turmeric).
- **Breakfast**: Smoothie bowl with fresh berries and seeds.
- **Lunch: Cucumber and Avocado Salad**
- **Dinner**: Grilled fish with steamed vegetables (transition meal).
- **Tip**: Ensure to drink plenty of water throughout the day.

Day 13:

- **Morning**: Lemon water.
- **Breakfast: Quinoa Breakfast Bowl with Mango and Avocado**
- **Lunch**: Fresh fruit salad with a variety of seasonal fruits.
- **Dinner: Sautéed Kale and Mushroom Bowl**
- **Tip**: Avoid snacking on processed foods, opt for nuts and seeds instead.

Day 14:

- **Morning**: Herbal tea (dandelion root).
- **Breakfast: Amaranth Porridge with Berries**
- **Lunch**: Mixed vegetable wrap with hummus.
- **Dinner: Roasted Butternut Squash and Avocado Salad**
- **Tip**: Practice deep breathing exercises or meditation to support stress management.

Summary of Week 2:

- **Daily Goals**: Replace most meals with Dr. Sebi-approved recipes, while allowing a few transition meals that are not strictly compliant.
- **Key Focus**: Incorporate more core alkaline foods like leafy greens, whole grains, and fresh fruits and vegetables.
- **Recipes Included**: Quinoa Breakfast Bowl with Berries and Nuts, Teff Porridge with Fresh Fruit, Chia Seed Pudding, Alkaline Breakfast Smoothie, Chickpea and Wild Rice Stuffed Bell Peppers, Amaranth and Vegetable Soup, Zucchini Noodles with Walnut Pesto, Cucumber and Avocado Salad, Quinoa Breakfast Bowl with Mango and Avocado, Sautéed Kale and Mushroom Bowl, Roasted Butternut Squash and Avocado Salad.
- **Lifestyle Changes**: Increase the intake of raw foods, reduce refined grains, stay hydrated, and incorporate stress management practices like deep breathing exercises or meditation.

Week 2 helps transition the diet further towards Dr. Sebi's guidelines, focusing on integrating core alkaline foods while still allowing some flexibility. This gradual shift supports the body in adapting to the new dietary habits and further enhancing detoxification.

Week 3: Deepening the Detox with Anti-Inflammatory Recipes

Goal: Fully eliminate non-compliant habits and meals, replacing all meals with Dr. Sebi-approved recipes. Focus on deepening the detox and enhancing overall well-being through strict adherence to Dr. Sebi's guidelines.

Day 15:

- **Morning**: Warm lemon water.
- **Breakfast: Sea Moss Smoothie**
- **Lunch: Spelt Pasta with Avocado Pesto**
- **Dinner: Chickpea and Wild Rice Stuffed Bell Peppers**
- **Tip**: Increase physical activity with daily walks or yoga.

Day 16:

- **Morning**: Herbal tea (peppermint).
- **Breakfast: Quinoa Breakfast Bowl with Berries and Nuts**
- **Lunch: Cucumber and Avocado Salad**
- **Dinner: Amaranth and Vegetable Soup**
- **Tip**: Practice mindfulness or meditation to enhance mental clarity.

Day 17:

- **Morning**: Herbal tea (Any Dr. Sebi-approved herb of choice; refer to the list)
- **Breakfast: Chia Seed Pudding**
- **Lunch: Sautéed Kale and Mushroom Bowl**
- **Dinner: Zucchini Noodles with Walnut Pesto**
- **Tip**: Focus on eating slowly and mindfully, chewing thoroughly.

Day 18:

- **Morning**: Fresh vegetable juice (cucumber, celery, and apple).
- **Breakfast: Alkaline Breakfast Smoothie**
- **Lunch: Roasted Butternut Squash and Avocado Salad**
- **Dinner: Baked Teff Falafel with Cucumber Mint Sauce**
- **Tip**: Increase water intake to at least 10 glasses a day.

Day 19:

- **Morning**: Herbal tea (any Dr. Sebi-approved herb of choice; refer to the list).
- **Breakfast: Quinoa Breakfast Bowl with Mango and Avocado**
- **Lunch: Teff Porridge with Fresh Fruit**
- **Dinner: Sautéed Kale and Mushroom Bowl**
- **Tip**: Avoid all processed foods, focusing on whole, natural ingredients.

Day 20:

- **Morning**: Lemon water.
- **Breakfast: Amaranth Porridge with Berries**
- **Lunch: Cucumber and Avocado Salad**
- **Dinner: Chickpea and Wild Rice Stuffed Bell Peppers**
- **Tip**: Engage in light exercise such as stretching or Pilates.

Day 21:

- **Morning**: Herbal tea (dandelion root).
- **Breakfast: Sea Moss Smoothie**
- **Lunch: Zucchini Noodles with Walnut Pesto**
- **Dinner: Amaranth and Vegetable Soup**
- **Tip**: Incorporate deep breathing exercises throughout the day to support detoxification.

Summary of Week 3:

- **Daily Goals**: Replace all meals with Dr. Sebi-approved recipes, fully eliminating non-compliant foods and habits.
- **Key Focus**: Deepen the detox by adhering strictly to Dr. Sebi's guidelines and incorporating more anti-inflammatory foods.
- **Recipes Included**: Sea Moss Smoothie, Quinoa Breakfast Bowl with Berries and Nuts, Cucumber and Avocado Salad, Amaranth and Vegetable Soup, Chia Seed Pudding, Sautéed Kale and Mushroom Bowl, Zucchini Noodles with Walnut Pesto, Roasted Butternut Squash and Avocado Salad, Baked Teff Falafel with Cucumber Mint Sauce, Quinoa Breakfast Bowl with Mango and Avocado, Teff Porridge with Fresh Fruit, Amaranth Porridge with Berries, Chickpea and Wild Rice Stuffed Bell Peppers.
- **Lifestyle Changes**: Increase physical activity, practice mindfulness, ensure thorough chewing, enhance hydration, avoid processed foods, and engage in light exercise and deep breathing exercises.

Week 3 solidifies the detox process by strictly following Dr. Sebi's dietary recommendations and integrating additional lifestyle changes to support and enhance the body's natural detoxification pathways.

Week 4: Establishing Long-Term Habits

Goal: Solidify long-term habits that support an alkaline lifestyle, including proper diet, sleep, rest, recreation, exercise, and other lifestyle practices. Continue with Dr. Sebi-approved recipes and introduce sustainable practices for lasting health.

Day 22:

- **Morning**: Warm lemon water.
- **Breakfast: Alkaline Breakfast Smoothie**

- **Lunch**: **Roasted Butternut Squash and Avocado Salad**
- **Dinner**: **Chickpea and Wild Rice Stuffed Bell Peppers**
- **Tip**: Ensure 7-9 hours of quality sleep each night. Establish a calming bedtime routine, such as reading or meditation.

Day 23:

- **Morning**: Herbal tea (peppermint).
- **Breakfast**: **Teff Porridge with Fresh Fruit**
- **Lunch**: **Cucumber and Avocado Salad**
- **Dinner**: **Amaranth and Vegetable Soup**
- **Tip**: Schedule regular physical activity, like 30 minutes of walking or yoga. Aim for consistency rather than intensity.

Day 24:

- **Morning**: Warm water with apple cider vinegar.
- **Breakfast**: **Chia Seed Pudding**
- **Lunch**: **Sautéed Kale and Mushroom Bowl**
- **Dinner**: **Zucchini Noodles with Walnut Pesto**
- **Tip**: Practice mindfulness or meditation daily to reduce stress. Try apps like Headspace or Calm if you need guidance.

Day 25:

- **Morning**: Fresh vegetable juice (cucumber, celery, and apple).
- **Breakfast**: **Quinoa Breakfast Bowl with Berries and Nuts**
- **Lunch**: **Roasted Butternut Squash and Avocado Salad**
- **Dinner**: **Baked Teff Falafel with Cucumber Mint Sauce**
- **Tip**: Spend time outdoors to reconnect with nature. Activities like walking, gardening, or simply sitting in a park can be beneficial.

Day 26:

- **Morning**: Herbal tea (any Dr. Sebi-approved herb of choice; refer to the list).
- **Breakfast**: **Sea Moss Smoothie**
- **Lunch**: **Zucchini Noodles with Walnut Pesto**
- **Dinner**: **Amaranth and Vegetable Soup**
- **Tip**: Prioritize hydration. Carry a water bottle and ensure you drink throughout the day.

Day 27:

- **Morning**: Lemon water.
- **Breakfast**: **Quinoa Breakfast Bowl with Mango and Avocado**
- **Lunch**: **Cucumber and Avocado Salad**
- **Dinner**: **Chickpea and Wild Rice Stuffed Bell Peppers**
- **Tip**: Reduce screen time, especially before bed. Aim for at least an hour of screen-free time before sleep to improve sleep quality.

Day 28:

- **Morning**: Herbal tea (dandelion root).
- **Breakfast**: **Amaranth Porridge with Berries**
- **Lunch**: **Sautéed Kale and Mushroom Bowl**
- **Dinner**: **Roasted Butternut Squash and Avocado Salad**
- **Tip**: Incorporate a hobby or activity that brings joy and relaxation, such as reading, painting, or playing a musical instrument.

Summary of Week 4:

- **Daily Goals**: Continue with Dr. Sebi-approved recipes, and integrate long-term lifestyle habits to support overall health and well-being.
- **Key Focus**: Establish sustainable habits for sleep, rest, recreation, exercise, and stress management.
- **Recipes Included**: Alkaline Breakfast Smoothie, Roasted Butternut Squash and Avocado Salad, Chickpea and Wild Rice Stuffed Bell Peppers, Teff Porridge with Fresh Fruit, Cucumber and Avocado Salad, Amaranth and Vegetable Soup, Chia Seed Pudding, Sautéed Kale and Mushroom Bowl, Zucchini Noodles with Walnut Pesto, Quinoa Breakfast Bowl with Berries and Nuts, Baked Teff Falafel with Cucumber Mint Sauce, Sea Moss Smoothie, Quinoa Breakfast Bowl with Mango and Avocado, Amaranth Porridge with Berries.
- **Lifestyle Changes**: Ensure quality sleep, regular physical activity, mindfulness practices, time outdoors, hydration, reduced screen time, and engaging in hobbies for relaxation.

Week 4 focuses on cementing the alkaline lifestyle by integrating comprehensive health and wellness practices, ensuring the habits formed during the detox plan become part of a sustainable, healthy lifestyle.

Week-by-Week Changes and Perceived Benefits

Week 1: Cleansing and Preparation

In the first week, your body begins to adjust to the reduction of problematic foods like caffeine, sugar, and processed items. Initially, you might experience mild withdrawal symptoms such as headaches or fatigue as your system clears out toxins. However, as you increase your water intake and introduce detoxifying drinks like lemon water and herbal teas, you'll notice your digestion starting to improve. Your body will begin to feel lighter, and bloating will reduce. Mentally, the transition may be challenging, but sticking to the plan will help you start feeling more energized and focused by the end of the week. This week sets the foundation for deeper detoxification and prepares your body for the transition to a more alkaline diet.

Week 2: Integrating Core Alkaline Foods

As you enter the second week, the integration of more Dr. Sebi-approved recipes and alkaline foods into your diet will become more noticeable. Your body will start to feel more balanced and energized. You'll likely experience an increase in vitality as your digestion improves further, and you may notice clearer skin and better hydration. Cravings for unhealthy foods will diminish, making it easier to stick to the plan. Mentally, you'll begin to feel more clarity and focus, as the nutrient-rich foods support better brain function. By the end of this week, you'll feel a significant reduction in inflammation and may notice improved joint flexibility and less muscle stiffness.

Week 3: Deepening the Detox with Anti-Inflammatory Recipes

In the third week, your body fully transitions to a Dr. Sebi-compliant diet, which accelerates the detoxification process. You will likely experience a marked improvement in your overall health. The anti-inflammatory properties of the foods will help reduce any chronic pain or discomfort, and you might feel a newfound sense of well-being. Energy levels will be higher, and you'll notice an improvement in your mood and mental sharpness. Physically, you may observe weight loss and a more toned appearance as your body sheds excess toxins and inflammation. Your digestive system will function optimally, resulting in regular bowel movements and reduced bloating. Mentally, you'll feel more grounded and emotionally balanced, as your body and mind sync with the alkaline lifestyle.

Week 4: Establishing Long-Term Habits

By the fourth week, the benefits of the detox plan will be fully apparent. Your body will have adapted to the new diet, and you'll find it easier to maintain these healthy eating habits. You'll feel consistently energized throughout the day, and your sleep patterns will improve, leading to more restful nights. With the incorporation of regular physical activity, mindfulness, and proper hydration, your overall fitness and mental health will reach new heights. You'll experience a sustained sense of mental clarity and emotional stability, making stress management more effective. Skin clarity, reduced bloating, and a leaner physique will be noticeable physical changes. By the end of this week, the habits you've formed will feel natural, setting you up for long-term health and wellness in alignment with Dr. Sebi's principles.

Through this transformative month, you'll witness significant improvements in both physical and mental health, laying the groundwork for a lifetime of balanced, alkaline living.

CHAPTER 6

20 Delicious and Nutritious Recipes

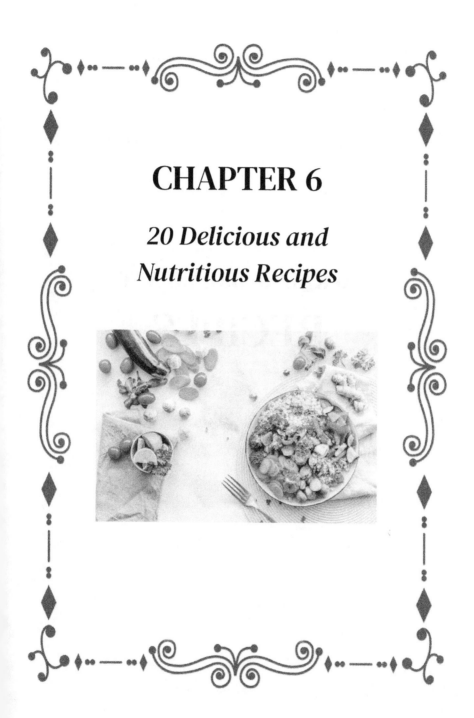

ALKALINE BREAKFAST
RECIPES

Quinoa Breakfast Bowl with Berries and Nuts

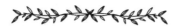

Prep time: 10 mins
Cooking time: 15 mins
Servings: 2

Ingredients:
- 1 cup cooked quinoa
- 1/2 cup fresh blueberries
- 1/2 cup fresh raspberries
- 1/4 cup chopped walnuts
- 1 tbsp agave syrup
- 1 tsp chia seeds

Directions:

1. **Prepare the Quinoa**: Rinse 1 cup of quinoa thoroughly under cold water to remove its natural bitterness. Cook the quinoa according to the package instructions, usually by bringing it to a boil in 2 cups of water and then simmering it for about 15 minutes until all the water is absorbed. Let the quinoa cool slightly.
2. **Combine Ingredients**: In a medium bowl, combine the cooked quinoa, fresh blueberries, fresh raspberries, and chopped walnuts. Drizzle with 1 tablespoon of agave syrup for natural sweetness.
3. **Mix and Serve**: Gently mix all the ingredients until well combined. Sprinkle 1 teaspoon of chia seeds on top for an extra boost of nutrients. Serve immediately and enjoy a nutritious, energizing breakfast.

Nutritional Facts: Calories 320; Fat 12g; Carbohydrates 44g; Proteins 8g; Cholesterol 0mg; Sodium 15mg; Potassium 390mg

Teff Porridge with Fresh Fruit

Prep time: 10 mins
Cooking time: 20 mins
Servings: 2

Ingredients:

- 1 cup teff
- 3 cups water
- 1 cup homemade walnut milk
- 1 tbsp agave syrup
- 1/2 cup sliced strawberries
- 1/2 cup blueberries
- 1/4 cup chopped walnuts
- 1 tbsp chia seeds

Directions:

1. **Rinse and Cook the Teff**: Rinse 1 cup of teff under cold water. In a medium saucepan, bring 3 cups of water to a boil. Add the rinsed teff, reduce the heat to low, cover, and let it simmer for about 15-20 minutes or until the water is absorbed and the teff is tender.
2. **Add Homemade Walnut Milk and Sweeten**: Stir in 1 cup of homemade walnut milk and 1 tablespoon of agave syrup. Continue to cook over low heat for an additional 5 minutes, stirring occasionally, until the porridge reaches your desired consistency.
3. **Serve with Fresh Fruit and Nuts**: Divide the cooked teff porridge into two bowls. Top each serving with 1/2 cup of sliced strawberries, 1/2 cup of blueberries, 1/4 cup of chopped walnuts, and 1 tablespoon of chia seeds. Serve warm for a nutritious and satisfying breakfast.

Nutritional Facts: Calories 380; Fat 14g; Carbohydrates 56g; Proteins 10g; Cholesterol 0mg; Sodium 15mg; Potassium 500mg

Chia Seed Pudding

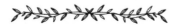

Prep time: 10 mins
Cooking time: 0 mins (plus overnight chilling)
Servings: 2

Ingredients:

- 1 cup homemade walnut milk
- 1/4 cup chia seeds
- 1 tbsp agave syrup
- Fresh berries for topping

Directions:

1. **Combine Ingredients**: In a medium bowl, whisk together 1 cup of homemade walnut milk, 1/4 cup of chia seeds, and 1 tablespoon of agave syrup.
2. **Chill Overnight**: Cover the bowl and refrigerate overnight, or for at least 4 hours, until the chia seeds have absorbed the liquid and the mixture has thickened to a pudding-like consistency.
3. **Serve**: Divide the chia seed pudding into serving bowls and top with fresh berries. This pudding is a healthy and satisfying snack or breakfast, rich in omega-3 fatty acids and fiber.

Nutritional Facts: Calories 200; Fat 10g; Carbohydrates 20g; Proteins 5g; Cholesterol 0mg; Sodium 40mg; Potassium 200mg

Quinoa Breakfast Bowl with Mango and Avocado

Prep time: 10 mins
Cooking time: 20 mins
Servings: 2

Ingredients:

- 1 cup quinoa
- 2 cups water
- 1 cup homemade hempseed milk
- 1 tbsp agave syrup
- 1 ripe mango, diced
- 1 avocado, diced
- 1/4 cup raw sunflower seeds
- 1 tbsp chia seeds

Directions:

1. **Cook the Quinoa**: Rinse 1 cup of quinoa under cold water. In a medium saucepan, bring 2 cups of water to a boil. Add the rinsed quinoa, reduce the heat to low, cover, and let it simmer for about 15 minutes or until the water is absorbed and the quinoa is tender.
2. **Add Homemade Hempseed Milk and Sweeten**: Stir in 1 cup of homemade hempseed milk and 1 tablespoon of agave syrup. Continue to cook over low heat for an additional 5 minutes, stirring occasionally, until the mixture is creamy.
3. **Serve with Fresh Fruit and Seeds**: Divide the cooked quinoa into two bowls. Top each serving with diced mango, avocado, 1/4 cup of raw sunflower seeds, and 1 tablespoon of chia seeds. Serve warm for a hearty and nutritious breakfast.

Nutritional Facts: Calories 400; Fat 18g; Carbohydrates 58g; Proteins 12g; Cholesterol 0mg; Sodium 10mg; Potassium 600mg

Spelt Pancakes with Berry Compote (Using Natural Leavening)

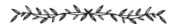

Prep time: 10 mins
Cooking time: 20 mins
Servings: 2

Ingredients:

- 1 cup spelt flour
- 1 cup homemade walnut milk
- 1 tbsp agave syrup
- 1 tbsp grapeseed oil
- 1/2 cup mixed berries (blueberries, raspberries, strawberries)
- 1/4 cup water
- 1 tbsp agave syrup for compote
- 1/4 cup aquafaba (liquid from cooked chickpeas) or 1 tsp natural yeast

Directions:

1. **Prepare the Pancake Batter**: In a medium bowl, mix 1 cup of spelt flour, 1 cup of homemade walnut milk, 1 tablespoon of agave syrup, 1 tablespoon of grapeseed oil, and 1/4 cup aquafaba (or 1 tsp natural yeast). Stir until the batter is smooth.
2. **Cook the Pancakes**: Heat a non-stick pan over medium heat. Pour 1/4 cup of batter onto the pan for each pancake. Cook until bubbles form on the surface, then flip and cook until golden brown on both sides. Repeat until all batter is used.
3. **Make the Berry Compote**: In a small saucepan, combine 1/2 cup of mixed berries, 1/4 cup of water, and 1 tablespoon of agave syrup. Cook over medium heat until the berries break down and the mixture thickens slightly, about 5-7 minutes.
4. **Serve**: Stack the pancakes on a plate and top with the warm berry compote. Serve immediately for a delicious and healthy breakfast.

Nutritional Facts: Calories 350; Fat 10g; Carbohydrates 58g; Proteins 10g; Cholesterol 0mg; Sodium 15mg; Potassium 400mg

Alkaline Breakfast Smoothie

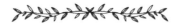

Prep time: 10 mins

Cooking time: 0 mins

Servings: 2

Ingredients:

- 1 cup homemade walnut milk
- 1/2 cup fresh kale
- 1/2 cup frozen blueberries
- 1/2 avocado
- 1 tbsp chia seeds
- 1 tbsp agave syrup

Directions:

1. **Prepare the Ingredients**: Gather all ingredients: 1 cup of homemade walnut milk, 1/2 cup of fresh kale, 1/2 cup of frozen blueberries, 1/2 of a ripe avocado, 1 tablespoon of chia seeds, and 1 tablespoon of agave syrup.
2. **Blend the Smoothie**: In a blender, combine the walnut milk, kale, blueberries, avocado, chia seeds, and agave syrup. Blend on high speed until smooth and creamy. The combination of avocado and walnut milk provides a rich, creamy texture, while the spinach and blueberries add nutrients and a vibrant color.
3. **Serve**: Pour the smoothie into glasses and serve immediately. This smoothie is packed with healthy fats, fiber, and antioxidants, making it a perfect energizing breakfast.

Nutritional Facts: Calories 220; Fat 12g; Carbohydrates 26g; Proteins 4g; Cholesterol 0mg; Sodium 70mg; Potassium 500mg

Amaranth Porridge with Berries

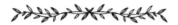

Prep time: 10 mins
Cooking time: 20 mins
Servings: 2

Ingredients:

- 1 cup amaranth
- 2 cups water
- 1/2 cup mixed berries (blueberries, raspberries, blackberries)
- 1 tbsp agave syrup

Directions:

1. **Cook the Amaranth**: Rinse 1 cup of amaranth under cold water. In a medium saucepan, bring 2 cups of water to a boil. Add the rinsed amaranth, reduce the heat to low, cover, and let it simmer for about 20 minutes or until the water is absorbed and the grains are tender.
2. **Sweeten the Porridge**: Stir in 1 tablespoon of agave syrup. Mix well to combine.
3. **Serve with Berries**: Divide the cooked amaranth porridge into bowls and top each serving with 1/2 cup of mixed berries. Serve warm. This porridge is a hearty and nutritious breakfast option that's rich in protein and fiber.

Nutritional Facts: Calories 290; Fat 4g; Carbohydrates 52g; Proteins 10g; Cholesterol 0mg; Sodium 5mg; Potassium 320mg

ANTI-INFLAMMATORY
LUNCHES AND
DINNERS

Spelt Pasta with Avocado Pesto

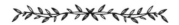

Prep time: 15 mins
Cooking time: 10 mins
Servings: 2

Ingredients:

- 2 cups spelt pasta
- 1 ripe avocado
- 1 cup fresh basil leaves
- 1/4 cup raw sunflower seeds
- 2 tbsp olive oil
- 1 tbsp lime juice
- Sea salt to taste

Directions:

1. **Cook the Pasta**: Bring a large pot of water to a boil. Add the spelt pasta and cook according to package instructions (usually about 10 minutes) until al dente. Drain and set aside.
2. **Prepare the Pesto**: In a food processor, combine the avocado, basil leaves, sunflower seeds, olive oil, lime juice, and sea salt. Blend until smooth and creamy.
3. **Mix and Serve**: Toss the cooked spelt pasta with the avocado pesto until well coated. Serve immediately and enjoy a nutritious, flavorful meal.

Nutritional Facts: Calories 450; Fat 22g; Carbohydrates 52g; Proteins 10g; Cholesterol 0mg; Sodium 10mg; Potassium 620mg

Chickpea and Wild Rice Stuffed Bell Peppers

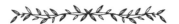

Prep time: 15 mins
Cooking time: 30 mins
Servings: 2

Ingredients:

- 2 large bell peppers
- 1 cup cooked wild rice
- 1 cup cooked chickpeas
- 1/2 cup chopped tomatoes
- 1/2 cup chopped kale
- 1 tbsp olive oil
- 1 tsp thyme
- Sea salt to taste

Directions:

1. **Prepare the Bell Peppers**: Preheat the oven to 375°F (190°C). Cut the tops off the bell peppers and remove the seeds and membranes. Set aside.
2. **Make the Filling**: In a large bowl, combine the cooked wild rice, chickpeas, chopped tomatoes, kale, olive oil, thyme, and sea salt. Mix well.
3. **Stuff and Bake**: Fill the bell peppers with the rice and chickpea mixture. Place them in a baking dish and cover with foil. Bake for 30 minutes, until the peppers are tender.
4. **Serve**: Allow the stuffed peppers to cool slightly before serving. Enjoy a hearty and healthy meal.

Nutritional Facts: Calories 300; Fat 10g; Carbohydrates 45g; Proteins 12g; Cholesterol 0mg; Sodium 20mg; Potassium 550mg

Amaranth and Vegetable Soup

Prep time: 10 mins
Cooking time: 20 mins
Servings: 2

Ingredients:
- 1/2 cup amaranth
- 4 cups vegetable broth
- 1 cup chopped zucchini
- 1/2 cup chopped kale
- 1 tbsp olive oil
- 1 tsp thyme
- Sea salt to taste

Directions:
1. **Cook the Amaranth**: In a medium pot, bring 4 cups of vegetable broth to a boil. Add the amaranth, reduce heat to low, and simmer for 15 minutes.
2. **Add Vegetables**: Stir in the chopped zucchini, and kale. Add the olive oil, thyme, and sea salt. Simmer for another 10 minutes, until the vegetables are tender.
3. **Serve**: Ladle the soup into bowls and serve warm. Enjoy a nutritious and comforting meal.

Nutritional Facts: Calories 220; Fat 8g; Carbohydrates 34g; Proteins 6g; Cholesterol 0mg; Sodium 15mg; Potassium 400mg

Zucchini Noodles with Walnut Pesto

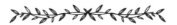

Prep time: 15 mins
Cooking time: 5 mins
Servings: 2

Ingredients:
- 2 large zucchinis, spiralized
- 1 cup fresh basil leaves
- 1/4 cup walnuts
- 2 tbsp olive oil
- 1 tbsp lime juice
- Sea salt to taste

Directions:
1. **Prepare the Zucchini Noodles**: Spiralize the zucchinis into noodles and set aside.
2. **Make the Pesto**: In a food processor, combine the basil leaves, walnuts, olive oil, lime juice, and sea salt. Blend until smooth.
3. **Mix and Serve**: Toss the zucchini noodles with the walnut pesto until well coated. Serve immediately for a fresh, raw meal.

Nutritional Facts: Calories 250; Fat 20g; Carbohydrates 16g; Proteins 5g; Cholesterol 0mg; Sodium 10mg; Potassium 600mg

Sautéed Kale and Mushroom Bowl

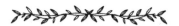

Prep time: 10 mins
Cooking time: 10 mins
Servings: 2

Ingredients:
- 4 cups chopped kale
- 1 cup sliced mushrooms
- 1 tbsp olive oil
- 1 tsp thyme
- Sea salt to taste

Directions:
1. **Heat the Oil**: In a large skillet, heat the olive oil over medium heat.
2. **Sauté the Vegetables**: Add the sliced mushrooms and cook for about 5 minutes, until they start to soften. Add the chopped kale and cook for another 5 minutes, stirring frequently.
3. **Season and Serve**: Sprinkle with thyme and sea salt. Serve warm as a nutritious side dish or a light main course.

Nutritional Facts: Calories 150; Fat 10g; Carbohydrates 12g; Proteins 4g; Cholesterol 0mg; Sodium 20mg; Potassium 550mg

Roasted Butternut Squash and Avocado Salad

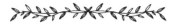

Prep time: 10 mins
Cooking time: 25 mins
Servings: 2

Ingredients:
- 2 cups diced butternut squash
- 1 avocado, diced
- 2 tbsp olive oil
- 1 tbsp lime juice
- 1/4 cup chopped cilantro
- Sea salt to taste

Directions:
1. **Roast the Squash**: Preheat the oven to 400°F (200°C). Toss the diced butternut squash with 1 tablespoon of olive oil and spread it on a baking sheet. Roast for 25 minutes, until tender and lightly browned.
2. **Prepare the Salad**: In a large bowl, combine the roasted butternut squash, diced avocado, remaining olive oil, lime juice, chopped cilantro, and sea salt. Toss gently to mix.
3. **Serve**: Serve the salad immediately for a fresh and flavorful dish.

Nutritional Facts: Calories 300; Fat 22g; Carbohydrates 26g; Proteins 3g; Cholesterol 0mg; Sodium 15mg; Potassium 700mg

Baked Teff Falafel with Cucumber Sauce

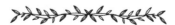

Prep time: 20 mins
Cooking time: 30 mins
Servings: 2

Ingredients:
- 1 cup teff flour
- 1 cup cooked chickpeas
- 1/4 cup chopped parsley
- 2 tbsp olive oil
- 1 tsp cumin
- Sea salt to taste

Cucumber Sauce:

- 1/2 cup chopped cucumber
- 1/2 cup homemade walnut milk
- 1 tbsp lime juice
- Sea salt to taste

Directions:
1. **Prepare the Falafel**: Preheat the oven to 375°F (190°C). In a food processor, combine the teff flour, cooked chickpeas, chopped parsley, olive oil, cumin, and sea salt. Blend until smooth.
2. **Form and Bake**: Shape the mixture into small balls and place them on a baking sheet lined with parchment paper. Bake for 30 minutes, turning halfway through, until golden brown.
3. **Make the Sauce**: In a blender, combine the chopped cucumber, homemade walnut milk, lime juice, and sea salt. Blend until smooth.
4. **Serve**: Serve the baked falafel with the cucumber sauce for dipping.

Nutritional Facts: Calories 350; Fat 16g; Carbohydrates 42g; Proteins 10g; Cholesterol 0mg; Sodium 20mg; Potassium 450mg

SNACKS AND
BEVERAGES

Sea Moss Smoothie

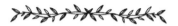

Prep time: 10 mins
Cooking time: 0 mins
Servings: 2

Ingredients:
- 2 tbsp sea moss gel
- 1/2 cup frozen mango
- 1 cup coconut water
- 1 tsp agave syrup

Directions:
1. **Prepare the Ingredients**: Ensure you have 2 tablespoons of prepared sea moss gel, which can be made by soaking and blending dried sea moss. Gather the frozen mango, coconut water, and agave syrup.
2. **Blend the Smoothie**: In a blender, combine the sea moss gel, 1/2 cup of frozen mango chunks, 1 cup of coconut water, and 1 teaspoon of agave syrup. Blend until the mixture is completely smooth and creamy.
3. **Serve**: Pour the smoothie into glasses and serve immediately. This smoothie is a refreshing, nutrient-packed snack or meal replacement.

Nutritional Facts: Calories 120; Fat 0g; Carbohydrates 28g; Proteins 1g; Cholesterol 0mg; Sodium 20mg; Potassium 280mg

Cucumber and Avocado Salad

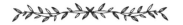

Prep time: 10 mins

Cooking time: 0 mins

Servings: 2

Ingredients:
- 1 large cucumber, diced
- 1 ripe avocado, diced
- 1/4 red onion, thinly sliced
- Juice of 1 lime
- 2 tbsp chopped cilantro
- Sea salt to taste

Directions:
1. **Prepare the Vegetables**: Dice the cucumber and avocado into bite-sized pieces. Thinly slice 1/4 of a red onion. Place all the vegetables into a large bowl.
2. **Dress the Salad**: Drizzle the juice of 1 lime over the vegetables. Add 2 tablespoons of chopped cilantro, and season with sea salt to taste.
3. **Toss and Serve**: Gently toss the salad to combine all the ingredients evenly. Serve immediately for a fresh, crisp, and creamy salad that's perfect as a snack or side dish.

Nutritional Facts: Calories 160; Fat 13g; Carbohydrates 12g; Proteins 2g; Cholesterol 0mg; Sodium 10mg; Potassium 600mg

Mango and Avocado Salsa

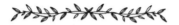

Prep time: 10 mins
Cooking time: 0 mins
Servings: 2

Ingredients:
- 1 ripe mango, diced
- 1 ripe avocado, diced
- 1/4 red onion, finely chopped
- Juice of 1 lime
- 2 tbsp chopped cilantro
- Sea salt to taste

Directions:
1. **Prepare the Ingredients**: Dice the mango and avocado, finely chop the red onion, and chop the cilantro.
2. **Combine Ingredients**: In a medium bowl, combine the diced mango, avocado, red onion, and chopped cilantro.
3. **Season and Serve**: Drizzle with the juice of 1 lime. Season with sea salt to taste. Gently toss to combine all the ingredients. Serve immediately with vegetable sticks or as a topping for salads. This salsa is a refreshing and nutritious snack, rich in vitamins and healthy fats.

Nutritional Facts: Calories 200; Fat 12g; Carbohydrates 25g; Proteins 2g; Cholesterol 0mg; Sodium 10mg; Potassium 500mg

Butternut Squash and Avocado Toast

Prep time: 10 mins
Cooking time: 15 mins
Servings: 2

Ingredients:
- 2 cups butternut squash, sliced into 1/4-inch-thick slices
- 1 ripe avocado, mashed
- 1 tbsp lime juice
- Sea salt to taste
- 1 tbsp hemp seeds

Directions:
1. **Prepare the Butternut Squash**: Preheat the oven to 400°F (200°C). Place the butternut squash slices on a baking sheet and bake for about 15 minutes, or until tender.
2. **Prepare the Avocado**: In a bowl, mash the avocado with lime juice and sea salt until smooth.
3. **Assemble the Toast**: Spread the mashed avocado onto the baked butternut squash slices. Sprinkle with hemp seeds.
4. **Serve**: Serve immediately as a nutritious and satisfying breakfast or snack.

Nutritional Facts: Calories 280; Fat 15g; Carbohydrates 33g; Proteins 3g; Cholesterol 0mg; Sodium 10mg; Potassium 700mg

Dr. Sebi's Herbal Tea

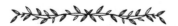

Prep time: 5 mins
Cooking time: 10 mins
Servings: 2

Ingredients:
- 2 cups water
- 1 tbsp dried burdock root
- 1 tbsp dried dandelion root
- 1 tbsp dried sarsaparilla root
- 1 tbsp dried ginger root

Directions:
1. **Prepare the Ingredients**: Measure out the dried burdock root, dandelion root, sarsaparilla root, and ginger root.
2. **Boil the Tea**: In a medium saucepan, bring 2 cups of water to a boil. Add the dried herbs to the boiling water and reduce the heat to low. Simmer for about 10 minutes.
3. **Strain and Serve**: After simmering, remove the tea from heat and strain out the herbs. Pour the herbal tea into cups and serve hot. This tea is known for its detoxifying and anti-inflammatory properties, making it an excellent beverage for overall health.

Nutritional Facts: Calories 10; Fat 0g; Carbohydrates 2g; Proteins 0g; Cholesterol 0mg; Sodium 5mg; Potassium 30mg

Alkaline Green Smoothie

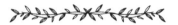

Prep time: 5 mins
Cooking time: 0 mins
Servings: 2

Ingredients:
- 2 cups fresh kale
- 1 cucumber, chopped
- 1 ripe avocado, peeled and pitted
- Juice of 1 lime
- 1-2 cups coconut water or alkaline water (adjust to desired consistency)
- Optional: 1 tablespoon ground flaxseeds or chia seeds

Directions:
1. **Prepare the Ingredients**: Wash the kale thoroughly. Peel and pit the avocado, and chop the cucumber.
2. **Blend the Ingredients**: In a blender, combine the fresh kale, chopped cucumber, and avocado.
3. **Add Lime Juice**: Squeeze the juice of one lime into the blender.
4. **Pour in Liquid**: Pour in 1-2 cups of coconut water or alkaline water, adjusting based on your desired consistency.
5. **Optional Nutrient Boost**: Optionally, add a tablespoon of ground flaxseeds or chia seeds for added nutrition.
6. **Blend Until Smooth**: Blend all the ingredients until smooth and creamy.
7. **Adjust Consistency**: If the smoothie is too thick, add more coconut water or alkaline water until you reach your desired consistency.
8. **Serve**: Pour the smoothie into glasses and serve immediately for a refreshing and alkalizing drink.

Nutritional Facts: Calories 150; Fat 10g; Carbohydrates 15g; Proteins 5g; Cholesterol 0mg; Sodium 50mg; Potassium 600mg

CHAPTER 7

Overcoming Challenges

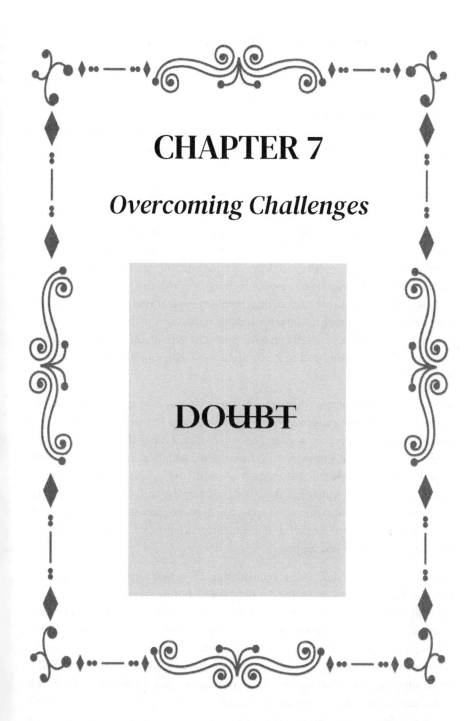

DOUBT

Common Pitfalls and How to Avoid Them

Navigating a dietary change, such as transitioning to the alkaline or anti-inflammatory diet, can be a transformative journey towards better health. However, it's not uncommon to encounter various challenges along the way. Understanding these common pitfalls and implementing effective strategies to overcome them is essential for maintaining dietary adherence and achieving long-term success.

One of the most prevalent challenges you face when adopting a new dietary regimen is the temptation to revert to old eating habits. This tendency is especially pronounced during times of stress or emotional upheaval when you may seek comfort in familiar comfort foods. Emotional eating can derail even the most well-intentioned dietary efforts, leading to feelings of guilt, frustration, and disappointment. To counteract emotional eating, it's crucial to cultivate mindfulness around eating habits. Mindful eating involves paying attention to the sensory experience of eating, such as the taste, texture, and aroma of food, as well as tuning into hunger and fullness cues. By practicing mindful eating, you can develop a deeper awareness of their eating patterns and make more conscious choices about when, what, and how much to eat.

In addition to mindfulness, identifying triggers that may lead to emotional eating is essential for developing alternative coping mechanisms. Stress, boredom, loneliness, and social pressures are common triggers for emotional eating. If you recognize these triggers early, you can preemptively address them with healthier coping strategies. Engaging in stress-relief activities such as meditation, yoga, or deep breathing exercises can help you manage stress without turning to food. Likewise, finding enjoyable hobbies, connecting with supportive friends or family members, or seeking professional support from a therapist or counselor can provide alternative outlets for emotional expression and support.

Another common pitfall when transitioning to a new dietary regimen is the misconception that healthy eating has to be bland, boring, or restrictive. Many of us fear that adopting a healthier diet means sacrificing flavor and enjoyment in their meals. This misconception can lead to feelings of deprivation and dissatisfaction, making it challenging to maintain long-term dietary adherence. To overcome this, emphasize the abundance of delicious and nutritious foods that can be enjoyed on an alkaline or anti-inflammatory diet, encouraging you to explore new recipes, experiment with different cooking techniques, and incorporate a variety of herbs, spices, and flavorful ingredients into your meals can help dispel this misconception.

In today's fast-paced world, many of us also struggle to find the time and resources necessary to plan, shop for, and prepare healthy meals consistently. Additionally, factors such as budget constraints and limited access to fresh, high-quality ingredients can further complicate efforts to adopt a healthier diet. However, with careful planning and resourcefulness, these obstacles can be overcome. Meal planning and preparation are indispensable components of maintaining a healthy diet. Try the following steps to successfully plan your meals:

1. The first step in meal planning is to allocate some time at the beginning of each week to plan out meals for the upcoming days. This involves considering factors such as dietary preferences, nutritional needs, and schedule constraints. Take stock of what ingredients are already on hand and what meals can be made with those ingredients, then you can minimize waste and make efficient use of your resources.

2. Creating a shopping list based on the planned meals is the next essential step. This helps you stay organized while grocery shopping and ensures you have all the necessary ingredients on hand when it comes time to cook. Including a variety of fruits, vegetables, whole grains, lean proteins, and healthy fats on the shopping list creates a well-rounded and nutritious diet.

3. Once the ingredients have been purchased, it's time to prepare them for use throughout the week. Batch cooking and meal prepping are highly effective strategies for saving time and effort in the kitchen. Batch cooking involves preparing large batches of food, such as soups, stews, or roasted vegetables, and portioning them out into individual servings for consumption later in the week. This not only saves time but also ensures that healthy options are readily available when hunger strikes.

4. Meal prepping takes batch cooking a step further by preparing entire meals or components of meals in advance. This may include cooking grains, chopping vegetables, marinating proteins, or assembling salads ahead of time. By having these components prepped and ready to go, you can quickly and easily assemble meals throughout the week, reducing the temptation to opt for less healthy convenience options.

In addition to meal planning and preparation, savvy shopping strategies can also help you make the most of your food budget while still enjoying nutritious meals. Shopping for seasonal produce can help save money, as seasonal items are often priced lower than out-of-season produce. Likewise, exploring alternative sources of fresh produce, such as farmers' markets, community-supported agriculture (CSA) programs, or online grocery delivery services, can provide access to high-quality ingredients at competitive prices.

While adopting a new dietary regimen like the alkaline or anti-inflammatory diet may present challenges, it's entirely achievable with the right mindset and strategies in place. With patience, perseverance, and a willingness to adapt, you can successfully navigate the challenges of dietary change and reap the numerous benefits of a healthier lifestyle.

Handling Social Situations and Dining Out

Social situations and dining out while sticking to a specific dietary regimen like the alkaline or anti-inflammatory diet can be tough. I understand, and you're not alone in feeling this way. But with a bit of planning, clear communication, and a flexible approach, you can enjoy social gatherings and restaurant outings without compromising your dietary goals.

One of the biggest challenges is not having control over the menu options. Restaurants and social events often have limited choices that may not fit your diet. Plus, there's the added pressure from friends and family to indulge in foods or drinks that you usually avoid. It can be tricky, but there're a few ways around it.

First, let's talk about planning ahead. If you're heading to a social event, consider reaching out to the host beforehand to ask about the menu. You could even offer to bring a dish that aligns with your diet. Most hosts will appreciate your proactive approach and be happy to accommodate you. When dining out, try to check the restaurant's menu online in advance. Look for dishes with alkaline-forming or anti-inflammatory ingredients like salads, grilled vegetables, lean proteins, and whole grains. And don't hesitate to ask the server if they can modify dishes to fit your needs. Many restaurants are more than willing to make adjustments like leaving out certain ingredients or switching sides.

When you talk about your dietary preferences, do it with confidence and kindness. Let your friends and the restaurant staff know that you're committed to your health and well-being. Framing your choices positively helps others understand and support you. It's also helpful to shift your focus from the food to the social aspects of the gathering. Enjoy the company of your friends and loved ones, engage in conversations, and participate in activities. This way, you won't feel as pressured by the food options.

Cravings can be tough, especially in social settings, so it's good to have a plan. Bring along healthy snacks or drinks that align with your diet. Practice mindful eating by savoring each bite and listening to your hunger and fullness cues to prevent overindulgence.

Remember, flexibility is key. It's important to prioritize your health, but it's also okay to have occasional deviations from your diet. Life is about balance, and one meal or snack won't derail your progress. Use these moments as opportunities to practice flexibility and resilience. Advocate for yourself and your dietary needs without hesitation. If you're unsure about the ingredients or preparation methods of a dish, ask the restaurant staff for more information. Your health and well-being are your top priorities, and it's okay to ask for what you need.

With planning ahead, communicating clearly, focusing on the social aspects of gatherings, and being flexible, you can stick to your dietary goals while enjoying social interactions and restaurant outings. Remember, it's okay to deviate from your regimen occasionally. Focus on making balanced choices that support your overall health and well-being.

FAQs and Troubleshooting Tips

50 Common Questions

1. **What is the Dr. Sebi diet, and who was Dr. Sebi?**
   The Dr. Sebi diet, developed by the late Dr. Sebi, is a plant-based diet focused on maintaining an alkaline environment in the body to promote overall health and prevent disease. Dr. Sebi, born Alfredo Darrington Bowman, was a Honduran herbalist and self-proclaimed healer who believed that an alkaline diet could detoxify the body and cure various ailments.

2. **What are the main principles of the Dr. Sebi diet?**
   The main principles of the Dr. Sebi diet are to consume natural, plant-based foods that are alkaline-forming and avoid acidic foods. This involves eating a variety of fruits, vegetables, nuts, seeds, and grains that maintain the body's natural pH balance. The diet emphasizes avoiding processed foods, animal products, and hybrid foods.

3. **What foods are allowed on the Dr. Sebi diet?**

   Allowed foods include fresh fruits like berries and apples, leafy greens like kale, vegetables like cucumbers and zucchini, nuts and seeds such as walnuts and chia seeds, and grains like quinoa and amaranth. Alkaline herbs and spices are also encouraged, along with plenty of water and natural teas.

4. **What foods are prohibited on the Dr. Sebi diet?**

   Prohibited foods include all animal products (meat, dairy, eggs), processed foods, refined sugars, artificial sweeteners, alcohol, caffeine, soy products, and hybrid or genetically modified foods. Vegetables like potatoes and carrots, and fruits like bananas are also avoided.

5. **How do I get started on the Dr. Sebi diet?**

   To get started, begin by gradually eliminating prohibited foods from your diet and incorporating more alkaline-forming foods. Plan your meals around Dr. Sebi-approved ingredients, and consider preparing some of his recommended recipes. Educate yourself on the foods to avoid and look for natural, whole food alternatives.

6. **Are there any potential side effects when starting the Dr. Sebi diet?**

   When starting the Dr. Sebi diet, some people may experience detox symptoms such as headaches, fatigue, or digestive changes as their bodies adjust. These symptoms are usually temporary and are a sign that the body is eliminating toxins. Staying hydrated and resting can help alleviate these symptoms.

7. **How long should I follow the Dr. Sebi diet to see results?**

   The time it takes to see results can vary depending on your starting point and health goals. Some people report feeling more energized and having improved digestion within a few weeks, while others may take longer to see significant changes. Consistency is key, and following the diet for several months can lead to more noticeable health improvements.

8. **Can I follow the Dr. Sebi diet if I have certain health conditions or dietary restrictions?**

   While many people with various health conditions have reported benefits from the Dr. Sebi diet, it's important to consult with a healthcare professional before making any significant dietary changes, especially if you have pre-existing health conditions or dietary restrictions. They can provide personalized guidance and ensure the diet is safe for you.

9. **What are the benefits of the Dr. Sebi diet?**

   The benefits of the Dr. Sebi diet include improved digestion, increased energy levels, weight loss, reduced inflammation, clearer skin, and overall better health. By focusing on nutrient-dense, natural foods, the diet supports the body's natural detoxification processes and helps maintain a balanced pH level.

10. **Are there any supplements recommended on the Dr. Sebi diet?**

    Yes, Dr. Sebi recommended various herbal supplements to complement the diet. These include Bio Ferro for iron and blood health, Viento for energy and detoxification, Chelation for removing toxins, and Sea Moss for a rich source of minerals. These supplements are designed to enhance the diet's effects and support overall health.

11. **How do I manage social situations and dining out while on the Dr. Sebi diet?**

    Managing social situations and dining out can be challenging, but planning ahead can help. Communicate your dietary preferences to hosts or restaurant staff, review menus in advance, and don't hesitate to ask for modifications. Bringing a dish to share at social gatherings and focusing on the social aspect rather than the food can also make it easier to stay on track.

    Is the Dr. Sebi diet suitable for children and pregnant women?

12. While the diet emphasizes natural, nutrient-dense foods, it may not meet all the nutritional needs of children and pregnant women. It's crucial to consult with a healthcare provider before making any dietary changes for these groups to ensure they receive adequate nutrition for growth and development.

13. **Can I exercise while following the Dr. Sebi diet?**

    Yes, you can exercise while following the Dr. Sebi diet. In fact, regular physical activity can complement the diet by promoting overall health and well-being. Ensure that you consume enough calories and nutrients to support your activity level, and listen to your body to avoid overexertion.

14. **How do I ensure I get enough protein on the Dr. Sebi diet?**

    The Dr. Sebi diet includes several plant-based sources of protein, such as nuts, seeds, leafy greens, and grains like quinoa and amaranth. Including a variety of these foods in your meals can help ensure you meet your protein needs. Additionally, Dr. Sebi-approved supplements can provide extra support if necessary.

15. **Are there any specific recipes or meal plans for the Dr. Sebi diet?**

    Yes, there are many Dr. Sebi-approved recipes and meal plans available online and in his published works. These resources provide a variety of meal ideas, from breakfast bowls and smoothies to soups, salads, and main dishes, all designed to help you follow the diet easily.

16. **How do I handle cravings for prohibited foods on the Dr. Sebi diet?**

Handling cravings can be challenging, but staying hydrated, eating regular meals, and ensuring you get enough nutrients can help. Find Dr. Sebi-approved alternatives to your favorite foods, and focus on the benefits of the diet to stay motivated. Mindfulness and distraction techniques can also be effective in managing cravings.

17. **What should I do if I experience detox symptoms while on the Dr. Sebi diet?**

If you experience detox symptoms, stay hydrated, rest, and give your body time to adjust. Eating a variety of nutrient-dense foods can help support the detox process. If symptoms persist or become severe, consult with a healthcare professional to ensure there are no underlying issues.

18. **How does the Dr. Sebi diet help with weight loss?**

The Dr. Sebi diet helps with weight loss by focusing on natural, whole foods that are low in calories and high in nutrients. This approach reduces the intake of processed and high-fat foods, which can lead to weight gain. The diet also promotes improved digestion and metabolism, further supporting weight loss efforts.

19. **Can I drink alcohol while following the Dr. Sebi diet?**

Alcohol is generally prohibited on the Dr. Sebi diet as it is considered acidic and can disrupt the body's pH balance. It's best to avoid alcohol to fully experience the benefits of the diet. Instead, opt for herbal teas, coconut water, or alkaline water as healthier beverage choices.

20. **How do I transition off the Dr. Sebi diet if needed?**

If you need to transition off the Dr. Sebi diet, do so gradually to avoid shocking your system. Slowly reintroduce non-approved foods in small amounts while monitoring how your body responds. Continue to focus on whole, natural foods and maintain some of the healthy habits you've developed to support your overall well-being.

21. **How do I prepare for starting the Dr. Sebi diet?**

Preparing for the Dr. Sebi diet involves educating yourself about the foods to include and avoid, planning your meals, and stocking your kitchen with approved ingredients. Begin by gradually eliminating prohibited foods from your diet to ease the transition. Having a support system, such as a friend or online community, can also help you stay motivated and informed.

22. **Are there any common mistakes to avoid on the Dr. Sebi diet?**

Common mistakes include not drinking enough water, not eating a variety of approved foods, and consuming too many processed "health" foods. It's essential to focus on whole, natural foods and stay hydrated to support detoxification and overall health. Additionally, avoid skipping meals or not consuming enough calories, as this can lead to nutrient deficiencies and energy loss.

23. **How can I find Dr. Sebi-approved products and ingredients?**

Dr. Sebi-approved products and ingredients can be found at health food stores, farmer's markets, and online retailers. Look for organic, non-GMO options to ensure the highest quality. Some specialty stores may carry specific Dr. Sebi-approved herbs and supplements. Reading labels and doing research can help you make informed choices.

24. **Can I follow the Dr. Sebi diet if I'm vegan or vegetarian?**

Yes, the Dr. Sebi diet is plant-based and naturally aligns with vegan and vegetarian lifestyles. It excludes all animal products, making it an excellent choice for those already following a vegan or vegetarian diet. Focus on the wide variety of approved fruits, vegetables, nuts, seeds, and grains to meet your nutritional needs.

25. **How does the Dr. Sebi diet support detoxification?**

The Dr. Sebi diet supports detoxification by emphasizing alkaline-forming foods that help maintain the body's natural pH balance. These foods are rich in vitamins, minerals, and antioxidants, which aid in removing toxins and promoting cellular health. Additionally, the diet encourages hydration, which helps flush out toxins through the kidneys and skin.

26. **Are there any cooking methods that are preferred on the Dr. Sebi diet?**

Preferred cooking methods include steaming, sautéing, baking, and grilling, as these methods preserve the nutrients in the food. Avoid deep-frying or using excessive oils and fats. Raw food preparation, such as salads and smoothies, is also encouraged to maximize nutrient intake.

27. **How important is hydration on the Dr. Sebi diet?**

Hydration is crucial on the Dr. Sebi diet as it aids in detoxification, digestion, and overall bodily functions. Drink plenty of water, herbal teas, and coconut water throughout the day to stay hydrated. Aim for at least 8-10 glasses of water daily, adjusting based on your activity level and needs.

28. **Can I eat out at fast-food restaurants on the Dr. Sebi diet?**

Fast-food restaurants typically offer limited options that align with the Dr. Sebi diet. It's best to avoid fast food and opt for dining establishments that offer fresh, whole food options. If you must eat out, choose simple salads or steamed vegetables and avoid dressings or sauces that may contain prohibited ingredients.

29. **What are some common myths about the Dr. Sebi diet?**

    Common myths include the belief that the diet lacks sufficient protein or essential nutrients, that it's too restrictive, or that it's a quick-fix solution. In reality, the Dr. Sebi diet can provide all necessary nutrients when properly planned, and it promotes long-term health rather than temporary results. Educating yourself and seeking credible information can help dispel these myths.

30. **How do I handle eating while traveling on the Dr. Sebi diet?**

    When traveling, plan ahead by researching restaurants that offer Dr. Sebi-approved options, packing snacks like nuts, seeds, and fruits, and carrying herbal teas or alkaline water. Staying flexible and making the best choices available can help you stick to the diet while on the go. Always keep hydration in mind and avoid processed foods.

31. **Is the Dr. Sebi diet expensive to follow?**

    The cost of the Dr. Sebi diet can vary depending on where you shop and the availability of approved foods. While some items like organic produce and specialty herbs may be more expensive, you can manage costs by buying in bulk, shopping at farmer's markets, and focusing on seasonal produce. Planning meals and reducing waste can also help keep expenses in check.

32. **How do I balance macronutrients on the Dr. Sebi diet?**

    Balancing macronutrients involves ensuring you get adequate amounts of carbohydrates, proteins, and fats from approved sources. Include a variety of fruits, vegetables, nuts, seeds, and grains in your meals. For example, quinoa and amaranth provide protein and carbs, while nuts and seeds offer healthy fats. This variety helps maintain nutritional balance and energy levels.

33. **Can I include fermented foods in the Dr. Sebi diet?**

    Fermented foods are generally not emphasized in the Dr. Sebi diet due to their potential acidity. However, some naturally fermented, minimally processed foods like sauerkraut or pickles might be acceptable in moderation. It's essential to focus on the core principles of the diet and avoid commercially processed fermented products that may contain additives or sugars.

34. **What are some quick and easy snack ideas for the Dr. Sebi diet?**

    Quick and easy snacks include fresh fruits like apples and berries, raw nuts and seeds, vegetable sticks with guacamole, sea moss gel smoothies, and homemade trail mix. These snacks provide convenient, nutrient-dense options that align with the diet's principles and keep you satisfied between meals.

35. **How can I deal with family members who are not supportive of my dietary choices?**

    Dealing with unsupportive family members can be challenging, but open communication is key. Explain your reasons for following the diet and the benefits you experience. Seek to educate and share information without being confrontational. Finding a supportive community, either online or locally, can provide additional encouragement and understanding.

36. **Are there any specific times of the day that are best for eating certain foods on the Dr. Sebi diet?**

    While the diet doesn't specify exact meal times, eating a balanced breakfast, lunch, and dinner with Dr. Sebi-approved foods can help maintain energy levels and support overall health. Consuming lighter meals in the evening and heavier meals earlier in the day can aid digestion and improve sleep quality. Listen to your body's hunger cues and adjust accordingly.

37. **Can I drink coffee or tea on the Dr. Sebi diet?**

    Coffee is prohibited on the Dr. Sebi diet due to its acidity and caffeine content. Instead, opt for herbal teas that are alkaline-forming and provide various health benefits. Teas like chamomile, ginger, peppermint, and dandelion root are excellent choices that align with the diet's principles and support overall well-being.

38. **What should I do if I feel hungry between meals on the Dr. Sebi diet?**

    If you feel hungry between meals, choose nutrient-dense snacks that align with the diet, such as fresh fruits, raw nuts, seeds, or vegetable sticks. Staying hydrated can also help manage hunger. Sometimes, thirst is mistaken for hunger, so drinking water or herbal tea can be beneficial.

39. **How does the Dr. Sebi diet affect my energy levels?**

    The Dr. Sebi diet can lead to increased energy levels due to its focus on nutrient-dense, alkaline-forming foods that support overall health. By avoiding processed foods and consuming natural ingredients, you provide your body with the vitamins and minerals it needs to function optimally. Many people report feeling more energized and less fatigued after transitioning to this diet.

40. **Are there any long-term studies on the effects of the Dr. Sebi diet?**

    Currently, there are limited scientific studies specifically on the Dr. Sebi diet. However, many of its principles align with well-researched dietary patterns, such as plant-based and alkaline diets, which have been shown to offer various health benefits. Anecdotal evidence and testimonials from followers suggest positive outcomes, but more research is needed to fully understand the long-term effects. Consulting healthcare professionals can provide additional insights and personalized advice.

41. **What is the role of fasting in the Dr. Sebi diet, and how should it be done?**
Fasting is an integral part of the Dr. Sebi diet as it helps the body detoxify and reset. Fasting can range from intermittent fasting, where you limit eating to a specific window each day, to longer fasts. Start with short fasting periods, gradually increasing the duration as your body adapts. Always ensure to stay hydrated and consult with a healthcare professional before undertaking longer fasts.

42. **Can the Dr. Sebi diet help with specific health issues like diabetes or hypertension?**
The Dr. Sebi diet, with its emphasis on natural, plant-based foods and avoiding processed items, can help manage conditions like diabetes and hypertension by improving blood sugar control and reducing blood pressure. However, it's crucial to consult with your healthcare provider to tailor the diet to your specific needs and ensure it's safe alongside any medications you might be taking.

43. **What is the significance of pH balance in the Dr. Sebi diet?**
The Dr. Sebi diet focuses on maintaining an alkaline pH balance in the body, as an alkaline environment is believed to promote better health and prevent disease. By consuming alkaline-forming foods and avoiding acidic ones, the diet aims to reduce inflammation, support detoxification, and enhance overall well-being.

44. **Are there any common detox symptoms to watch out for?**
Common detox symptoms include headaches, fatigue, digestive changes, and mild flu-like symptoms. These occur as your body eliminates toxins. Staying hydrated, getting plenty of rest, and eating a variety of nutrient-rich foods can help manage these symptoms. If they persist or become severe, consult with a healthcare professional.

45. **How can I make sure I am getting enough vitamins and minerals on the Dr. Sebi diet?**
To ensure you're getting enough vitamins and minerals, focus on eating a diverse range of approved fruits, vegetables, nuts, seeds, and grains. Incorporating supplements like sea moss gel, which is rich in essential minerals, can also help. Consulting with a nutritionist or dietitian can provide personalized guidance and prevent deficiencies.

46. **What are some good substitutes for common prohibited foods?**

For common prohibited foods like dairy, use homemade walnut milk or hempseed milk. Replace meat with protein-rich grains like quinoa and legumes such as chickpeas. Use agave syrup instead of refined sugar and swap white rice with amaranth or wild rice. Finding these alternatives can make the transition smoother and keep meals enjoyable.

47. **How do I deal with weight fluctuations on the Dr. Sebi diet?**

Weight fluctuations can be normal as your body adjusts to the new diet. Focus on consistent, nutrient-dense eating and avoid processed foods. Regular physical activity and staying hydrated can also help stabilize your weight. If weight fluctuations continue or cause concern, consult with a healthcare professional.

48. **Can the Dr. Sebi diet improve skin health, and how?**

Yes, the Dr. Sebi diet can improve skin health due to its emphasis on nutrient-rich, alkaline-forming foods. These foods help reduce inflammation and provide essential vitamins and antioxidants that support healthy skin. Many followers report clearer, more radiant skin after adhering to the diet.

49. **What are the best ways to prepare and store Dr. Sebi-approved foods?**

Preparing Dr. Sebi-approved foods involves using methods like steaming, sautéing, baking, and grilling to preserve nutrients. Store fresh produce in the refrigerator, and keep grains, nuts, and seeds in airtight containers in a cool, dry place. Batch cooking and freezing meals can also save time and ensure you always have compliant foods on hand.

50. **How can I stay motivated to stick with the Dr. Sebi diet?**

Staying motivated involves setting clear health goals, tracking your progress, and celebrating small victories. Surround yourself with a supportive community, whether it's friends, family, or online groups. Continually educate yourself about the benefits of the diet and remind yourself of the positive changes you've experienced. Maintaining a variety of delicious and satisfying meals can also keep you engaged and committed.

Quick Troubleshooting Tips for the Dr. Sebi Diet

1. **Experiencing withdrawal symptoms?** Stay hydrated and rest; symptoms are temporary.

2. **Seeing no results yet?** Be consistent and patient; it may take several weeks to notice changes.

3. **Have pre-existing health conditions?** Consult with a healthcare professional before starting.

4. **Cravings for prohibited foods?** Stay hydrated, eat regular meals, and find Dr. Sebi-approved alternatives.

5. **Social gatherings and dining out?** Plan ahead, communicate your dietary needs, and focus on the social aspect.

6. **Traveling while on the diet?** Research restaurants in advance, pack snacks, and stay hydrated.

7. **Facing family resistance?** Communicate openly and educate them about your dietary choices.

8. **Struggling with meal planning?** Use Dr. Sebi-approved recipes and meal plans to stay organized.

9. **Protein intake concerns?** Include a variety of approved nuts, seeds, leafy greens, and grains.

10. **Feelings of hunger between meals?** Opt for nutrient-dense snacks like fruits, nuts, and seeds.

11. **Exercise and diet balance?** Ensure you consume enough calories and nutrients to support your activity level.

12. **Managing restaurant meals?** Review the menu beforehand and ask for modifications to fit your diet.

13. **Cost concerns?** Buy in bulk, shop at farmer's markets, and plan meals to reduce waste.

14. **Hydration importance?** Drink at least 8-10 glasses of water daily to support detoxification.

15. **Maintaining energy levels?** Stick to nutrient-dense, natural foods to avoid fatigue.

16. **Navigating fast food?** Avoid fast food; choose simple salads or steamed vegetables if necessary.

17. **Reducing refined grains?** Replace with whole grains like quinoa and amaranth.

18. **Incorporating more raw foods?** Add fresh salads and raw vegetables to your meals.

19. **Transitioning off the diet?** Reintroduce non-approved foods gradually while monitoring your body's response.

20. **Starting the diet?** Educate yourself about allowed and prohibited foods, and plan meals accordingly.

21. **Fasting guidance?** Start with short fasting periods and gradually increase duration; stay hydrated.

22. **Managing diabetes or hypertension?** Consult with a healthcare provider to tailor the diet to your needs.

23. **Understanding pH balance?** Focus on consuming alkaline-forming foods to maintain your body's pH balance.

24. **Preventing nutrient deficiencies?** Eat a diverse range of approved foods and consider supplements if necessary.

25. **Substituting prohibited foods?** Use approved alternatives like homemade walnut milk, quinoa, and agave syrup.

26. **Handling weight fluctuations?** Focus on consistent, nutrient-dense eating and regular physical activity.

27. **Improving skin health?** Eat nutrient-rich, alkaline-forming foods to reduce inflammation and support skin health.

28. **Preparing and storing foods?** Use steaming, baking, and grilling; store properly to maintain freshness.

29. **Staying motivated?** Set clear goals, track progress, and engage with a supportive community.

30. **Addressing protein intake?** Incorporate a variety of plant-based protein sources like nuts, seeds, and grains.

31. **Handling social pressure?** Frame your dietary choices positively and seek understanding from others.

32. **Staying hydrated?** Prioritize drinking plenty of water, herbal teas, and coconut water throughout the day.

CHAPTER 8

Beyond the 28-Day Plan

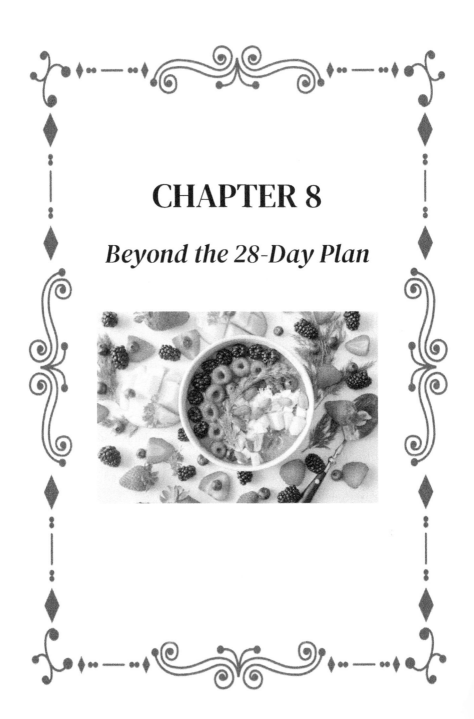

M aintaining an alkaline and anti-inflammatory lifestyle beyond the initial 28-day plan is essential for long-term health and well-being. This chapter delves into various strategies and considerations for sustaining this lifestyle over time.

Maintaining an Alkaline and Anti-Inflammatory Lifestyle

Consistency is paramount when it comes to maintaining an alkaline and anti-inflammatory lifestyle. While the initial 28-day plan may provide a jumpstart, it's crucial to integrate the principles of alkaline and anti-inflammatory eating into everyday life. This involves making conscious choices to prioritize whole, nutrient-dense foods while minimizing processed and inflammatory ones. Meal planning and preparation take center stage when trying to establish this consistency. They are invaluable tools for maintaining an alkaline and anti-inflammatory lifestyle. Take the time to plan out meals for the week, create shopping lists, and prepare ingredients in advance to streamline the cooking process and make it easier to stick to a healthy eating plan. Batch cooking and meal prepping are effective strategies for preparing large batches of food ahead of time and portioning them out for easy grab-and-go meals throughout the week. Additionally, shopping for seasonal, budget-friendly ingredients and exploring alternative sources of fresh produce, such as farmers' markets or community-supported agriculture (CSA) programs, can help you make the most of their food budget while still enjoying nutritious and satisfying meals.

In addition to dietary habits, other lifestyle factors play a significant role in maintaining alkaline and anti-inflammatory balance. Regular physical activity, adequate sleep, stress management, and mindfulness practices all contribute to overall well-being. Incorporating these practices into daily life supports the body's natural detoxification processes and reduces inflammation. Finding enjoyable forms of exercise, such as walking, yoga, or swimming, can make it easier to stay active consistently. Similarly, incorporating stress-reducing activities like meditation, deep breathing exercises, or spending time in nature can help manage stress levels and promote relaxation. There's also the social aspect of things, as we've mentioned several times before. Stay connected with a supportive community to maintain motivation and accountability—other people who were able to successfully transition into the Dr. Sebi diet. Whether through online forums, support groups, or social media communities, sharing experiences, challenges, and successes with like-minded you can provide encouragement and inspiration along the journey. Engaging with others who share similar health goals can offer valuable support and camaraderie, making it easier to stay on track with healthy habits.

If you're new to this diet—or new to lifestyle changes in general—you'll find yourself slinking away to old habits in the face of life's unplanned stresses, which is perfectly natural. Flexibility and adaptability are essential traits when it comes to maintaining an alkaline and anti-inflammatory lifestyle. While it's important to have a plan in place, life often throws unexpected curveballs that may require adjustments to dietary and lifestyle habits. Being flexible and open to change allows you to navigate these challenges gracefully and find solutions that work for them. Whether it's adapting recipes to accommodate dietary restrictions, finding creative ways to stay active during travel, or managing stress in challenging situations, being adaptable allows you to maintain their health and well-being in any circumstance. Our bodies and circumstances change, so what worked initially may need modification down the road. Regularly check in with yourself and evaluate how dietary and lifestyle choices are impacting overall health and well-being allows you to make informed decisions about how to proceed. This may involve experimenting with different foods, routines, or strategies to find what works best for individual needs and preferences. So, remain flexible and open to experimentation to find the approach that best suits your unique needs and preferences.

Advanced Tips and Techniques

1. Fine-Tuning Alkaline and Anti-Inflammatory Eating:

While the basics of alkaline and anti-inflammatory eating involve prioritizing whole, nutrient-dense foods and minimizing processed and inflammatory ones, advanced practitioners may seek to fine-tune their approach for optimal results. This may involve experimenting with different ratios of macronutrients (carbohydrates, fats, and proteins), exploring specific dietary protocols such as intermittent fasting or cyclical ketogenic diets, or incorporating targeted supplementation to address individual needs. Consulting with a knowledgeable healthcare professional or registered dietitian can provide personalized guidance and support in navigating these advanced dietary strategies.

2. Exploring Functional Foods and Nutraceuticals:

Functional foods and nutraceuticals are foods or food components that offer additional health benefits beyond basic nutrition. These may include superfoods like spirulina, chlorella, or wheatgrass, which are rich in chlorophyll and other phytonutrients with potent alkalizing and anti-inflammatory properties. Similarly, certain herbs, spices, and botanical extracts such as turmeric, ginger, boswellia, and green tea contain bioactive compounds that can help modulate inflammation and support overall health. Integrating these functional foods and nutraceuticals into the diet can provide additional support for maintaining alkaline and anti-inflammatory balance. But this comes with a caveat: While the ingredient may have overarching health benefits, they may not always align with Dr. Sebi's principles, so it is up to you to decide whether you want a puritan approach or a hybrid approach.

3. Stress Reduction and Mind-Body Practices:

Stress reduction and mind-body practices are integral components of an alkaline and anti-inflammatory lifestyle. Advanced practitioners may explore a variety of techniques to promote relaxation, resilience, and emotional well-being. This may include practices such as mindfulness meditation, yoga, tai chi, qigong, breathwork, or guided imagery, all of which have been shown to reduce stress and support overall health. Incorporating these practices into daily life can help you better manage stress, enhance emotional balance, and promote a sense of inner peace and well-being, something we all can benefit from.

4. Detoxification Strategies:

Advanced practitioners may explore various detoxification protocols to support the body's natural detoxification processes and promote elimination of toxins. This may include periodic fasting or cleansing regimens, targeted supplementation with liver-supportive herbs and nutrients, or incorporating specific detoxifying foods and beverages into the diet. It's important to approach detoxification with caution and under the guidance of a qualified healthcare professional, as certain protocols may not be appropriate for everyone as well as keeping in mind that every supplement may not comply with strict Dr. Sebi principles.

5. Sleep Optimization:

Optimizing sleep is critical for overall health and well-being and is often overlooked in discussions about alkaline and anti-inflammatory living. Advanced practitioners may prioritize sleep hygiene practices to ensure restorative and restful sleep. This may include creating a consistent sleep schedule, establishing a relaxing bedtime routine, optimizing sleep environment (such as minimizing exposure to blue light and creating a cool, dark, and quiet sleep environment), and addressing underlying sleep disorders or disturbances. Quality sleep is essential for supporting immune function, hormonal balance, cognitive function, and overall vitality, so it's one of our top recommendations if you want to go all in on this lifestyle.

Continuing Education and Resources

Now that you've reached the end of this elementary tome on Dr. Sebi's philosophy, how do you keep on growing? Continuing education and resources play a crucial role in supporting you on your journey towards maintaining an alkaline and anti-inflammatory lifestyle. One of the most effective ways to deepen knowledge and understanding of Dr. Sebi nutrition is through formal education and courses. There are numerous online and in-person programs available, ranging from basic nutrition courses to advanced certifications in functional medicine, integrative nutrition, or holistic health coaching. These programs provide comprehensive education on the principles of alkaline and anti-inflammatory eating, as well as practical tools and strategies for implementing these dietary approaches in everyday life. Additionally, many courses offer ongoing support, community forums, and resources to help participants stay engaged and motivated throughout their learning journey.

Check out the following resources if you're interested in this learning path:

1. Dr. Sebi's Nutritional Guide and Herbology

A specialized course focusing on Dr. Sebi's nutritional guidelines, including the approved and prohibited foods, herbal remedies, and their applications for health and healing.

- **Format**: Online
- **Website**: Dr. Sebi's Cell Food
- **Ideal for**: Individuals interested in a deep dive into Dr. Sebi's specific recommendations and herbal practices.

2. Holistic Health Coaching Certification

This program offers a broad education in holistic health, covering nutrition, lifestyle coaching, and the integration of various dietary philosophies, including the alkaline diet.

- **Format**: Online/In-person
- **Website**: Institute for Integrative Nutrition
- **Ideal for**: Those looking to become certified health coaches with a comprehensive understanding of holistic and integrative health practices.

3. Functional Medicine and Nutrition

An advanced program that delves into the principles of functional medicine, the role of nutrition in health and disease, and how to implement an anti-inflammatory diet.

- **Format**: Online/In-person
- **Website**: The Institute for Functional Medicine
- **Ideal for**: Healthcare practitioners and advanced learners interested in the scientific and practical aspects of nutrition.

4. Herbal Medicine and Nutrition

This course explores the use of herbs in nutrition and health, emphasizing Dr. Sebi's recommended herbs and their benefits.

- **Format**: Online
- **Website**: The Herbal Academy
- **Ideal for**: Individuals interested in the medicinal use of herbs in conjunction with an alkaline diet.

5. Mind-Body Nutrition Certification

Focuses on the connection between diet, mental health, and overall well-being. It includes principles of alkaline nutrition and stress management techniques.

- **Format**: Online
- **Website**: Mind Body Green
- **Ideal for**: Those looking to understand the holistic connection between nutrition and mental health.

If the course route is not your cup o' tea and you prefer something in solitude, books and publications are valuable resources to expand your knowledge of alkaline and anti-inflammatory nutrition. There are countless books available on these topics, ranging from introductory guides to advanced scientific texts written by experts in the field. Reading books allows you to delve deeper into specific areas of interest, gain insights from different perspectives, and access practical tips and recipes for incorporating alkaline and anti-inflammatory foods into their diet. A quick Amazon search on Dr. Sebi will offer you great recommendations. Additionally, subscribing to health and wellness magazines, newsletters, and online publications can provide ongoing inspiration, education, and updates on the latest research and trends in nutrition and wellness.

If you're interested in general health and fitness, attending health and wellness events, such as workshops, seminars, conferences, and retreats, can be an enriching experience for you to deepen your understanding of alkaline and anti-inflammatory living. These events provide opportunities to learn from leading experts in the field, participate in hands-on workshops and cooking demonstrations, connect with like-minded individuals, and immerse oneself in a supportive and inspiring environment. Additionally, many events offer practical tools and strategies for implementing healthy lifestyle changes, as well as opportunities for personal growth, reflection, and renewal.

Lastly, for those with a flair for a personalize and supervised approach, health coaching and support can be invaluable for on your journey towards maintaining an alkaline and anti-inflammatory lifestyle. Working with a qualified health coach or nutritionist can provide you with personalized support, tailored recommendations, and actionable steps for achieving their health goals. Health coaches can help you identify barriers to success, develop strategies for overcoming challenges, and create sustainable lifestyle changes that support long-term health and vitality. Additionally, many health coaches offer ongoing support, accountability, and motivation to help you stay on track and achieve lasting results.

So, continuing learning and seeking to maintain an alkaline and anti-inflammatory lifestyle. By investing in ongoing learning, connecting with supportive communities, attending health and wellness events, participating in online courses and webinars, and working with qualified health professionals, you can deepen your knowledge, expand your skills, and receive the support and guidance needed to achieve your health and wellness goals. With access to a wealth of resources and support networks, you can cultivate a vibrant, balanced, and resilient state of health that supports a thriving life.

BONUS EXTRA!!!

Scan the QR CODE

and Get Your **Dr. Sebi's Alkaline and Anti-Inflammatory Diet Transformation for Beginners Audiobook** and **Dr. Sebi's 7-Day Full-Body Detox Plan** -
All Straight into Your Email!!

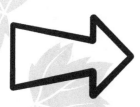  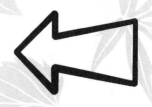

As SPAM Filters Are Pretty Crazy These Days...
...WHITELIST this Email Address!

info@greenessencepublishing.com

In This Way, Your Bonus Will Appear in the Main Folder of Your INBOX and They Will Not Be Buried Along With Other Advertisements in Your PROMOTION/SPAM Folder.

HERE IS HOW TO DO IT:
From Android Smartphone/Tablet
Open the Contacts App;
In the lower right corner, tap + (Add);
Enter the name and email address and then tap Save.

From iPhone/iPad
Open the Contacts App;
In the upper right corner, tap + (Add);
Enter the name and email address and then tap Finish.

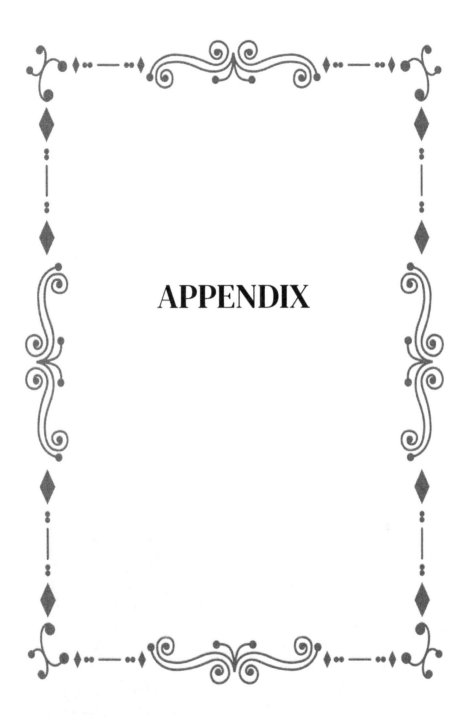

APPENDIX

Glossary of Terms

Alkaline Diet: A diet that emphasizes foods that increase the body's alkalinity, such as fruits, vegetables, nuts, and seeds, and discourages acidic foods like meat, dairy, and processed foods.

Anti-Inflammatory Diet: A diet designed to reduce inflammation in the body, often including foods rich in antioxidants and omega-3 fatty acids, such as fruits, vegetables, nuts, seeds, and fatty fish.

Bio Ferro: An herbal supplement formulated by Dr. Sebi to boost iron levels, support blood health, and improve energy and circulation.

Chelation: A process and a specific herbal compound aimed at removing heavy metals and toxins from the body, enhancing overall organ function.

Detoxification: The process of removing toxins from the body, often supported by specific diets, herbal supplements, and adequate hydration.

Electrical Foods: Foods that are natural, non-hybrid, and high in energy, believed by Dr. Sebi to support cellular health and vitality.

Fasting: Abstaining from all or certain types of food or drink for a period, believed to help the body detoxify and reset.

Mucus-Free Diet: A diet that avoids foods contributing to mucus production, such as dairy and processed foods, to promote overall health.

Natural Spring Water: Water from natural springs, recommended by Dr. Sebi for its purity and mineral content, supporting overall hydration and detoxification.

Nutrient-Dense Foods: Foods that are high in vitamins, minerals, and other essential nutrients relative to their calorie content.

Phytonutrients: Naturally occurring compounds in plants that have health-promoting properties, such as antioxidants, which help protect the body from damage.

Plant-Based Diet: A diet consisting primarily of foods derived from plants, including vegetables, fruits, nuts, seeds, oils, whole grains, legumes, and beans.

Viento: An herbal supplement created by Dr. Sebi, designed to provide natural energy, support mental clarity, enhance physical performance, and aid in detoxification.

Resource List

Books:

- "Dr. Sebi's Alkaline and Anti-Inflammatory Diet" by Gabrielle F. Wimmer
- "Dr. Sebi: The Man Who Cures AIDS, Cancer, Diabetes, and More" by Beverly Oliver
- "The Alkaline Cure: The Amazing 14 Day Diet and Cleanse" by Dr. Stephan Domenig

Websites:

- [Dr. Sebi's Official Website](https://drsebiscellfood.com)
- [Alkaline Foods List](https://www.alkalinefoods.net)
- [The Anti-Inflammatory Diet](https://www.healthline.com/nutrition/anti-inflammatory-diet-101)

Online Courses:

- "Plant-Based Nutrition" by eCornell
- "Herbal Medicine for Everyone" by The Herbal Academy

Support Groups and Forums:

- Facebook Groups dedicated to Dr. Sebi's diet and lifestyle
- Reddit communities focused on alkaline and anti-inflammatory diets

Herbal Supplement Stores:

- Dr. Sebi's Cell Food
- Mountain Rose Herbs
- Gaia Herbs

Documentaries and Videos:

- "Urban Kryptonite: African Roots, Foreign Diseases" (Documentary featuring Dr. Sebi)
- YouTube channels focused on plant-based diets and natural health

References and Further Reading

1. Books and Articles:

- "How Not to Die: Discover the Foods Scientifically Proven to Prevent and Reverse Disease" by Dr. Michael Greger
- "The Plant Paradox: The Hidden Dangers in 'Healthy' Foods That Cause Disease and Weight Gain" by Dr. Steven R. Gundry
- "The China Study: The Most Comprehensive Study of Nutrition Ever Conducted" by T. Colin Campbell and Thomas M. Campbell II

2. Scientific Journals:

- "Journal of Plant-Based Medicine"
- "Journal of Nutritional Biochemistry"
- "American Journal of Clinical Nutrition"

3. Research Papers:

- "Diet and inflammation" by Monica Bullon et al., published in Journal of Clinical Periodontology
- "Antioxidant and Anti-Inflammatory Activities of Various Dietary Plants Extracts" by M. Sharif et al., published in Journal of Food Science

4. Online Databases:

- PubMed (for peer-reviewed articles on nutrition and herbal medicine)
- Google Scholar (for a broad range of academic papers and articles)

By utilizing this appendix, readers can deepen their understanding of Dr. Sebi's dietary theories, find additional resources to support their journey, and access further reading to expand their knowledge on alkaline and anti-inflammatory lifestyles.

RECIPES INDEX